Praise for Totally CPAP

"It's a breath of fresh air to hear an acclaimed surgeon advocate for CPAP. We can now all breathe better and sleep better with another valuable and insightful book from Dr. Steven Park, my friend and colleague."

—Barry Krakow, M.D.
Author of *Sound Sleep, Sound Mind*

"Dr. Park's new book is a comprehensive book on CPAP that's easy to read and filled with practical advice. I highly recommend it."

—Avram R. Gold, MD
Medical Director, Stony Brook
University Sleep Disorders Center

"I have had the pleasure of working with Dr. Park to treat his PAP patients for more than a decade. His passion for finding the best possible treatment outcomes for his patients is clear and his depth of knowledge about PAP therapy makes this book an incredible resource for anyone using a PAP or interested in learning more about it."

—Chip Smith
President, Restoration Medical Supplies

"Dr. Park's logical step-by-step guide to troubleshooting CPAP problems will be a welcome and valuable resource for anyone who uses CPAP for sleep. It's an easy to understand book and it's rare to find a doctor with so much insight concerning the struggles mask users can come across – and he offers a workable solution for all of them! If there's such a thing as a holistic sleep physician and surgeon, Dr. Park is it. I highly recommend this book."

—**Kath Hope**
Founder & CEO of
Hope2Sleep Charity

"This book is a useful addition to the consumer literature on successfully treating sleep-disordered breathing."

—**Edward Grandi**
Former Executive Director of the
American Sleep Apnea Association

"I've been a sleep apnea patient for about 14 years now, wearing a CPAP mask every night. However, I have received more 'understanding' of what that is, how it happens, what helps/hurts breathing and information on the entire issue from Dr. Park. I have followed him online, and joined in some of the discussions he has with experts. This is a good, central source of 'cutting-edge' knowledge about apnea."

—**Marty Wilson**

"We CPAP users are very fortunate to have someone of Dr. Park's stature available to us in what otherwise is a 'desert' of help. His knowledge and willingness to share it is a blessing."

—**Ginny Edmundso**

"I've only just begun CPAP treatment and I already see a marked difference in my health, rest and ability to focus and function at work and at home. It is no exaggeration to say that Dr. Park's diagnosis and skill have changed, and perhaps saved, my life. Thank you."

—**Michael O'Neill**

Totally CPAP

Totally CPAP

A SLEEP PHYSICIAN'S GUIDE
TO RESTORING YOUR SLEEP
AND RECLAIMING YOUR LIFE

• • •

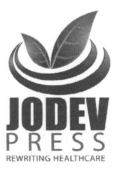

JODEV
PRESS
REWRITING HEALTHCARE

Steven Y. Park MD

For information about this title or to order other books and/or electronic media, please contact:

Jodev Press, LLC
91 Wood Avenue, Suite #1
Ardsley, NY 10502
www.JodevPress.com

ISBN: 0980236746
ISBN number: 9780980236743
Printed in the United States of America
Book cover design by: Liana Moisescu

Dedicated to all my patients and the online community who struggle tirelessly to achieve better sleep with CPAP.

I learned more from you than all the textbooks combined.

"Then the Lord God formed a man from the dust of the ground and breathed into his nostrils the breath of life, and the man became a living being."

—Genesis 2:7

Table of Contents

Foreword

• • •

I HAVE KNOWN DR. PARK for about 10 years and have personally been on the receiving end of the generous help he freely gives to those with sleep-disordered breathing, despite his own busy work schedule. His previous book, website, podcasts and presence in the sleep community make us wonder what his own secret is for all the energy he obviously has... oh I forgot... it's because he follows his own good sleep hygiene advice!

Dr. Park's previous book, *Sleep Interrupted*, gives real insight into the causes of sleep-disordered breathing, and now that he has written his new book, *Totally CPAP*, we have the 'total' package delivered by one of the most highly respected doctors working in the field of sleep medicine. I personally know many patients who are now able to have a much better quality of life, thanks to the resources and knowledge he has provided regarding the still largely overlooked sleep-disordered breathing condition, upper airway resistance syndrome (UARS).

Totally CPAP is now aimed at many of the same people who actually learned or suspected that they were living (suffering) with an undiagnosed sleep-breathing condition, through Dr. Park's first book, *Sleep Interrupted*. Of course, he will also come to the rescue of the many people out there who may be struggling with their therapy – and will give them a better quality of life once a few hiccups are addressed!

As the founder of the Hope2Sleep Charity, who deals every day with all the necessary support to help people cope with sleep-disordered breathing problems, I can say that it is rare to find a doctor who diagnoses patients AND has the answers for the many problems people living with these conditions face. As I have previously said, Dr. Park is the *total* package and his own patients are lucky to have him as their physician. However, those who can't see him in person can still benefit from his expertise by reading both of his books. I cannot rate them highly enough—in fact, our charity sells his first book so that people outside the USA can benefit from Dr. Park's educational materials. This latest book leaves no stone unturned regarding the issues so many people face. I would go so far as to say that *Totally CPAP* would do well in the hands of every sleep doctor and sleep tech to help them understand how they can support their own patients even more.

Dr. Park has an amazing ability to understand the frustrations and needs of people living with sleep-disordered breathing, and obviously works very hard to find viable solutions. On top of this, he also writes in layman's terms, so that even the sleepiest person can easily absorb the very information that could be the solution for them to live healthier and more energized lives, and just as importantly, to gain safe and comfortable sleep!

Best Wishes for Good Sleep,

Kath Hope, Founder & CEO of
Hope2Sleep Charity
www.hope2sleep.co.uk

Preface

· · ·

Why I Had to Write This Book

Sleep doctors will insist that there's nothing better than continuous positive airway pressure (CPAP), and for many of you, it works like a dream. However, for some of you, the thought of using CPAP gives you panic attacks. Others struggle to use the machine on a nightly basis. Some of you are even able to use it regularly, but your sleep quality has yet to improve.

You may also be frustrated with too much conflicting information on the Internet. Or perhaps your doctor isn't helpful – or even familiar – with the difficulties of using CPAP. Quite frankly, except for some rare exceptions, our healthcare system is generally quite lacking in terms of 'customer service.'

Although there are some very knowledgeable and passionate medical professionals out there, going through different components of sleep apnea care (medical, testing, dental, equipment, surgical) in different locations or institutions can be a challenging task to navigate. You also have to deal with information overload online.

These are the reasons why I had to write this book.

Why Should You Trust Me?

In my day job, I'm an academic otolaryngologist (ear, nose and throat surgeon), board certified in both otolaryngology and sleep medicine. I see and treat thousands of sleep apnea patients every year.

My main mission is to help those of you with sleep apnea get the sleep you need to have the life you want. Over the past 15 years, I've been on a quest to educate sleep apnea sufferers like you on how to breathe better so that you can sleep better. With my first book, *Sleep, Interrupted: A physician reveals the #1 reason why we're so sick and tired*, I educated thousands of people who were frustrated with their constant fatigue and chronic illnesses, helping them to recognize that these issues may be due to a breathing problem, rather than a sleep problem.

I also saw many people with sleep apnea either being misled on the Internet, or falling through the cracks despite good intentions by various healthcare professionals. In order to educate and teach more people about this condition, I started a blog eight years ago, which you can read at doctorstevenpark.com. My blog was voted one of the "Best Sleep Disorders Blogs of 2016" by Healthline.com, Best of Doctor's Websites 2106 by Pacific Medical Training, and a "Top 10 online influencer of sleep discussion" by Sharecare.com.

In addition, over the last 10 years, I've been invited to speak all over the country to educate other sleep physicians and healthcare professionals on how to better manage and treat their patients who have sleep apnea.

I don't say all of this to impress you, but rather to impress upon you how passionate I am about my mission.

Despite a wealth of helpful information being available, in general, I find that OSA sufferers like you can find all this information to be challenging to navigate. Oftentimes, you can feel alone and isolated, even with well-meaning family members or medical providers, as they simply may not understand. This is a common theme that I see again and again—people with the right tools and knowhow who want to help and patients who are looking for the right kind of help, but there seems to be a major disconnect between these two groups.

I hope that this book can bridge this gap in communication and understanding, not only between patients and healthcare providers, but also between successful and unsuccessful CPAP users.

Unfortunately, with recent changes in our healthcare system, I'm seeing more and more patients falling through the cracks with CPAP therapy. Today, it's not enough to rely on your healthcare providers for your most important medical problems. You must take an active part – if not take control – in demanding the highest quality medical care and service.

But You're a Surgeon!

So why is an ENT surgeon giving you advice for your CPAP? As a physician and surgeon, my main priority is to "first do no harm." This maxim means to err on the side of what's best for the patient and not what's best for me. Of course, I love what I do—there's no greater joy for me than surgically helping my patients breathe better during the day, and especially at night while they sleep. However, what I love more is to help OSA sufferers like you succeed in getting your OSA treated *without* surgery—whether or not it involves me.

For some of you, by the time you've come to see me, you've pretty much tried everything else. This also means that you're quite desperate and are willing to go to extremes to get better. Many of you have lost your jobs, are on disability, divorced, have had two heart attacks and are on multiple medications, or are seeing 10 different doctors, etc. etc. You're hoping that there's another way that will finally help you sleep better.

If the impression of your first experience is negative, it colors the next time you encounter a similar episode. Multiply that experience over and over and there's bound to be serious negative psychological consequences as a result. It is the same way for people with OSA. If you have a bad experience with CPAP as your first initial treatment for OSA, it's going to be that much harder for you to try another mode of therapy, or maybe you won't want to try anything else at all. That's why patients often let sleep apnea linger until it devastates every area of their life. By the time they do take action, it's often too late.

That's why I wrote this book. In a way, I'm trying to turn back the clock for all of you—back to what I could have done to help you many years ago when you were first diagnosed with sleep apnea and tried CPAP. I want to show what you could have gone through to make it easier, and how different life would have been for you, if a DME provider, doctor, or sleep study center held your hand through the process. I want to share years of sage advice that I have collected from my hundreds of encounters with other successful CPAP users, despite similar obstacles. Basically, I want to give you the second chance that you never had.

WHY YOU MUST READ THIS BOOK

Having sleep apnea and using CPAP is often like putting together a puzzle with a thousand different pieces, but without a complete picture of what all the pieces should look like. Of course, it's possible that if you took the time and patience to work through it, you might eventually be able to piece things together. Yet, how much faster and more easily could you complete the puzzle if someone gave you the complete picture from the start? Well, this book is meant to provide you with the sum total of that complete picture!

In fact, by reading and applying the concepts I share with you in this book, you'll bypass months or even years of frustration, self-doubt, and anguish that many first-time and experienced CPAP users face when dealing with and navigating our dysfunctional healthcare system. Instead, by figuring out what the beginning, middle and end look like, you'll be able to take full control of your own therapy and health. You'll no longer have to play 'healthcare hopscotch,' jumping from one specialist to another without getting any real resolutions to your problems. Nor will you fall victim to the paralysis by analysis that many CPAP users face by having so many choices without a guide to help them arrive at the right solution.

By learning to take control of your own CPAP success, you'll be taking the difficult but necessary steps to counter the detrimental effects that untreated sleep apnea can have on your life. Who knows—by sleeping better, you might be able to reclaim that energy and vitality you had before sleep apnea. Hopefully, you'll feel better than you ever did before!

Are you ready to take control? If so, then let's get started!

Introduction

• • •

"The defining factor for success is never
resources—it's resourcefulness."

—ANTHONY ROBBINS

YOU WERE JUST DIAGNOSED WITH obstructive sleep apnea and were given a machine and mask (continuous positive airway pressure, CPAP) to use at night in order to sleep better. You go home happily, looking forward to a great night's sleep for the first time in years. However, the first night is a miserable experience. You try again for the next few nights, but your sleep quality actually seems worse than before you started using CPAP. You make multiple trips to your sleep laboratory and call your equipment company a dozen times for help, but nothing seems to work. After four weeks of misery, you give up and resign yourself to living life in a fog, with no energy or joy whatsoever. If you are one of the thousands of people who are struggling with CPAP, this book is for you.

Successful companies like GE and Toyota use proven systems to achieve consistently good results. Likewise, with CPAP, there are proven systems that work well when applied properly. Unfortunately, many people are given CPAP haphazardly, with little education, support, or follow-up. On the other hand, some patients refuse to give CPAP an honest try, giving up much too early.

If you have been successful at using CPAP, then you don't need to read this book. I wrote this book mainly for those of you who struggle with CPAP, or those who are ready to give up altogether. Countless times every day, patients ask me what they can do to get CPAP to work for them. This book is my answer to all of you who are struggling to find the answers to help you get a great night's sleep and start enjoying life again.

> **Start Here**
>
> For a more thorough review of obstructive sleep apnea, and to learn why you and so many millions of others around you have obstructive sleep apnea, refer to my first book *Sleep, Interrupted: A physician reveals the #1 reason why so many of us are sick and tired.* Another good resource to start with is an article I wrote on the basics of obstructive sleep apnea (doctorstevenpark.com/osa).

If you're completely new to CPAP, this book may save you months or years of struggling and frustration. If you already have the basic knowledge and experience of using CPAP, and want to start troubleshooting right away, then skip the introductory chapters and begin at Chapter 4. Even if you find one simple tip that helps you sleep better with CPAP, then I've accomplished my goal. However, I hope that you'll get many significant insights and inspiration by reading this book.

As you are probably aware, obstructive sleep apnea (OSA) is a condition where you frequently stop breathing throughout the night due to overly relaxed muscles in your throat. Untreated OSA has been strongly associated with an increased risk of high blood pressure, diabetes, heart disease, heart attack, stroke, memory problems, cancer and even death.

It's been widely observed that untreated severe OSA can lower your life expectancy by about 20 years. Despite reliable studies showing that you can prevent this from happening by using CPAP, many patients give up after trying CPAP, or even worse, do nothing at all. In my experience, whenever I twist a reluctant patient's arm to try CPAP, about 10 to 20% end up loving it.

WHY CPAP?

I use the term CPAP to describe any type of machine that blows positive air pressure into your nose and/or mouth to keep your airway open, preventing you from choking repeatedly throughout the night. Despite the cold and technical terms used to describe CPAP, I've had some patients describe it in very endearing terms like "my honey" or "Pappy."

CPAP has been around since its invention by Dr. Colin Sullivan in the early 1980s. There are a number of other non-prescription, over-the-counter options that people can try (nasal dilator strips, chin straps or mouth guards), which do help some people, but overall, studies have shown very limited results. Of the three major formal medical options for treating sleep apnea (CPAP, dental devices, surgery), CPAP has the longest track record and the most research-based studies supporting its use.

Since the 1980s, CPAP has matured to become the standard of care for sleep apnea by the medical community. It's commonly referred to as the 'gold standard' treatment option for obstructive sleep apnea. Despite all the arguments for and against CPAP, it's an option that all sleep apnea sufferers should seriously consider, especially if you have severe sleep apnea. However, you'll only see these benefits if you use it! This book will give you proven steps that can significantly raise the chances that you'll not only be able to use CPAP, but also feel the benefits. If others have been successful, why not give CPAP a try for yourself?

What You'll Learn from This Book

Through my website, teleseminars and live events, I noticed a recurring trend—there are about 20 to 30 common questions about CPAP that my readers and patients ask me over and over again. In this book, I've done my best to answer these questions, as well as provide you with the latest information and technological advances on CPAP by constantly scanning medical research journals, along with attending and presenting at various sleep conferences What this book will offer you is my 15+ years of medical insight from treating and managing sleep apnea for tens of thousands of patients, and more importantly, everything that I've learned by listening to you through my live events and online activities.

Whether you're new to CPAP, have been struggling on CPAP for years, or if someone you love is having trouble with CPAP, then this book is for you.

By reading this book, you'll learn:

* The ONE thing you can do to increase CPAP use every night by up to five hours (Chapter 8).
* A step-by-step, easy-to-follow strategy that will significantly improve your chances of success with CPAP, not to mention getting higher quality sleep (Chapter 9).
* The top 15 most common problems that the average OSA sufferer has when beginning CPAP therapy and how you can avoid them altogether (Chapter 6).
* Why CPAP can sometimes worsen and not improve your sleep if you don't take this ONE piece of advice (Chapter 6).
* How to find and choose the right mask for you (Chapter 2).
* How you can find, access and even develop your own online support community for continued CPAP advice from other users (Chapter 10).

And finally,

* What you can do if CPAP doesn't work, even if you're using it religiously (besides throwing it in the trash!) (Chapter 10).

How to Use This Book

There are many good books on CPAP, ranging from academic textbooks to easy-to-digest e-books. In this book, I've pulled together all the pearls of wisdom from many of these sources and compiled a practical guide to help you navigate your journey while using CPAP. Frankly, this book should be included with every new CPAP machine. Better yet, it should be required reading as soon as someone is diagnosed with sleep apnea, but long before you try CPAP.

CPAP may not be the answer for everyone, but many people who give up on it barely scratch the surface of all the troubleshooting steps that can radically change your life for the better. Day after day, I consistently hear from patients how drastically improved their lives have been since starting CPAP, including having more energy, more creativity, less brain fog, and actually enjoying life again.

My goal with this book is to give you a better chance at succeeding with CPAP and having the opportunity to tell others that CPAP has changed your life.

Tony Robbins, the personal success guru, once gave a TED talk where he talked about what it takes to be successful in any area of life. He asked the audience why they failed to achieve something significant in their lives. The responses included lack of money, time, leadership, intellect, knowledge and technology. Even Al Gore, who was in the audience, claimed that he didn't have enough Supreme Court justices to get elected. Robbins noted that all these things relate to a lack of resources, but that the defining factor is actually a lack of resourcefulness.

In this book, I'm going to give you all the necessary tools to help you significantly increase your chances of not only being able to use CPAP, but also to sleep better with it. However, it will be your *resourcefulness* to apply these concepts that will ultimately determine whether or not you're successful. You need to be willing to be creative and to constantly improvise and experiment, just like the many successful CPAP users' stories that I'll be sharing with you throughout this book.

The first section (Chapters 1-3) will go over the basic fundamentals of CPAP devices, masks and insurance issues.

The second section (Chapters 4-8) is the most practical part of the book. I will cover the proper mindset issues and the latest research on what makes people stick with CPAP and eventually see significant benefits. I also address the most common problems that people have with CPAP, along with other miscellaneous issues that frequently arise in my practice. I also include a chapter on how to un-stuff your stuffy nose, which is critical for optimal CPAP use.

The last section (Chapters 9-10) will lay out a seven-day, step-by-step approach to starting CPAP that can significantly boost your chances of not only using CPAP, but also sleeping much better with it. In Chapter 10, I'll end with a brief discussion of your options if you've already given CPAP everything you've got. It won't give you every option available, but it will definitely give you a solid perspective of the most scientifically proven options outside of CPAP.

Remember, it's a universal principle that nothing happens until something moves. In the case of CPAP, that movement has to come from you and no one else. This is because it's you – not your physician, CPAP equipment vendor or spouse – who risks losing the most if CPAP fails.

You'll only need a few hours to read this book, but the investment will be worth it, namely because I've seen this advice work countless times. Not a week goes by without an email from a former patient thanking me for "giving them their life back." Patients often tell me on their follow-up visits how much weight they've lost (a 55-year-old accountant once told me that he'd lost 40 pounds since using CPAP!), or how they finally have enough energy back to enjoy precious time with their children.

My favorite moments are when some of my most stubborn and reluctant patients (usually built like NFL linebackers) come back for their follow-up visits and almost knock me over with their bear hugs, wide grins spread across their faces and tears of joy streaming down. They're thankful that I, like any good coach, helped them do what they initially couldn't do alone.

Of course, success doesn't happen overnight, but trust me, the few hours you invest in reading this book will pay infinite dividends. If you can achieve success with CPAP, just imagine what other areas of your life will improve with better sleep and better health. All of these example patients I just mentioned have done it. Now what about you? All it takes is a single step forward and the rest will fall into place. The real question is... Are you ready to trust me?

DISCLAIMER AND TRANSPARENCY

You'll commonly see or hear physicians with disclaimers stating that what's mentioned in their book, podcast or program should not be taken as medical advice, and that you should talk to your physician before making any changes to your diet or health regimen. I include the same disclaimer here in this book, as well as on my website doctorstevenpark.com.

However, if you've ever read any of my books or blog posts, or listened to my podcasts, then you know that I hold nothing back. I call it as I see it.

As with many medical conditions, there are many different competing treatment options, and sleep apnea is no exception. I will include relevant medical research when needed, but I've found that even with respected medical studies, you must take the advice with a grain of salt. You have to use common sense and decide for yourself whether or not you want to try one or more of my recommendations. By all means, please consult multiple physicians about the problem, or about my proposed solutions. I guarantee that you'll get conflicting opinions.

I've also placed links to resources either on my website or externally. With the exception of Amazon (where I get a very small commission if you buy anything), I have no financial arrangements with any other websites or organizations.

Everything You Wanted to Know About CPAP

• • •

"Your next step is simple. You are the first domino."

—GARY KELLER

AUTHOR, *THE ONE THING: THE SURPRISINGLY SIMPLE TRUTH BEHIND EXTRAORDINARY RESULTS*

CHAPTER 1

Mastering the Fundamentals of CPAP

• • •

*"I discovered early on that the player who
learned the fundamentals...is going to have a
much better chance of succeeding..."*

—John Wooden
Legendary UCLA Basketball Coach

Jason is a 55-year-old teacher who has struggled over the past few years with waning energy and constant forgetfulness that has been gradually getting worse. He came to see me for his severe snoring, which was keeping his wife awake. I suggested a sleep study, which revealed that Jason had moderately severe obstructive sleep apnea. Within the first week after using CPAP at home, he told me that he had gotten his life back.

This is only one of hundreds of CPAP success stories that I hear from patients every year. Some people take to CPAP like fish to water, while others struggle through a period of adjustment. Some, unfortunately, can't use CPAP no matter how hard they try.

What I've observed over the years is that the people who end up succeeding tend to have similar characteristics: they go through the fundamentals systematically, and have strong, crystal-clear reasons for why they need to succeed. It's not just about troubleshooting to make CPAP work. It's about being able to spend quality time with your spouse or children. It's about being able to focus and be just as productive at work as you used to be. For some people, it's about not dying of a heart attack like your father did at age 55 from untreated obstructive sleep apnea.

John Wooden, the legendary UCLA basketball coach, stressed the importance of developing the fundamentals of any endeavor if you want to achieve success. This chapter will cover the basic fundamentals of CPAP, so that you'll be better prepared to handle the challenges and obstacles that will likely arise when you start using CPAP.

CPAP Basics

CPAP stands for 'continuous positive airway pressure.' A gentle flow of positive air pressure is passed from the machine to a mask that fits snugly over your nose, or over your nose and mouth. The mask is typically made of air-cushioned padding and relies on straps around your head. The pressure level is usually calibrated during a second sleep study (CPAP titration), once a sleep apnea diagnosis is made. During the titration study (sleep study using CPAP), air pressure through the mask is gradually raised to eliminate apneas and hypopneas. This is the most effective way of quickly calibrating the pressure. A machine will then be ordered for you that is already set at this optimum pressure.

An apnea during a sleep study is defined as totally obstructed breathing that lasts for more than 10 seconds. Hypopneas also have to last more than 10 seconds, but with more than 30% obstructed breathing, where your brain waves show that you are waking up, or if your oxygen level is dropping more than 3-4%. To receive a diagnosis of obstructive sleep apnea, you'll need at least 15 apneas or hypopneas per hour. You can also receive a sleep apnea diagnosis if you have five or more apneas or hypopneas every hour, but only if you have any of the following: excessive daytime sleepiness, impaired cognition, mood disorders, insomnia, high blood pressure, heart disease, heart attack, or stroke. Most insurance providers follow Medicare's coverage guidelines for obstructive sleep apnea.

There are a number of different positive airway pressure machines, as well as different types of masks. In most cases, positive air pressure is delivered along with heated humidification to prevent nasal dryness and congestion. Note that these are not devices that deliver oxygen. Since OSA is a problem with obstructed breathing at night, positive air pressure from the machine allows you to breathe normally again, but delivering higher levels of oxygen when you're not able to breathe is not a good idea.

APAP

An APAP, or automatic positive airway pressure machine, uses a computer-controlled algorithm to continually and automatically adjust the air pressure throughout the night. Your doctor will set the upper and lower pressure limits. The machine will start off at the lowest pressure, but will gradually raise the pressure until all your apneas and hypopneas are gone. It constantly monitors your breathing and makes adjustments accordingly. Your pressure needs may change from hour to hour, or from day to day, depending on whether you have nasal congestion due to allergies, your sleep stages, or if your sleep position changes.

Some studies have shown that APAP may prevent more apneas and hypopneas and use lower average pressures, which can be more comfortable for patients. Different manufacturers use different algorithms, so you may have different experiences. APAP machines can also operate in straight CPAP mode. In other words, once the optimal pressure is recorded (from data that the machine provides), it can be set at that constant pressure for a while, and then re-calibrated using the automatic setting every few months or years on an as-needed basis.

You may be thinking by now that if APAP is so good, why doesn't everyone just use APAP? One reason is the cost. APAP is more expensive. Medicare (which insurance companies generally follow) sets reimbursement rates for all CPAP and APAP devices at only one level. Whether the doctor orders a CPAP or APAP machine, it's paid at one flat rate. Bi-level devices and above are reimbursed at about twice that of CPAP and APAP. Most insurance providers may not allow for any of the more advanced models unless you've tried straight CPAP or APAP first.

Now, with more insurance companies requiring home sleep testing, patients who are diagnosed with OSA are given APAP directly, bypassing the sleep lab entirely. While there are pros and cons to this approach, it's clearly a cost-saving measure. Paying a few hundred dollars more for an APAP machine probably saves more money than the traditional models (in-lab pressure calibration and CPAP), despite the less than ideal circumstances.

While some people prefer the automatic models over straight constant pressure, others do prefer the latter. The reason for this may be that the constant rising and lowering of the pressures can cause some people to awaken, especially if they are light sleepers. I've had people go from both CPAP to APAP and APAP to CPAP with success. This finding is in line with studies showing that overall, there is no significant objective or subjective difference between CPAP, bi-level, or automatic devices.[1-3] Just like any scientific studies, they reported overall averages, but didn't take into account individual variations. Sleep physicians will tell you that about 1/3 prefer CPAP, 1/3 prefer bi-level machines, and 1/3 like APAP. This may explain why some patients prefer one over the other. Ultimately, the only way to know which you'll like is to try each one. However, this may be challenging, since insurance companies generally want you to start with straight CPAP, or for home-based testing, APAP.

Therefore, depending on your insurance requirements and your particular situation, you may not have a choice of which type of PAP machine you start off with. My suggestion is to start with what's initially recommended, but make sure that you've gone through all the troubleshooting steps in these CPAP chapters before you consider switching to a new machine. For example, if you're having mask leak issues, switching from CPAP to APAP won't make a difference.

The algorithms for APAP, although they are fairly accurate, are not perfect. Different manufacturers do have different algorithms. Certain machines will be better at detecting more subtle obstructive events, such as respiratory event-related arousals (RERAs) or flow limitations. RERAs are similar to hypopneas, but don't meet the >30% lowered airflow criteria. Flow limitations are very subtle levels of obstructed breathing that are picked up on the nasal airflow channel and that show up as flattened airflow signals lasting less than 10 seconds. At times, this can cause your brain to wake you up to varying degrees.

Bi-level PAP

A bi-level machine provides two pressures: a higher level during inhalation and a lower level during exhalation. This makes breathing out easier, especially if your pressure is very high. BiPAP is a trade name from one of the major CPAP companies (Respironics), so from now on, I'll use the term bi-level. This technology tracks and responds to your breathing patterns during inhalation and exhalation.

ADAPTIVE SERVO-VENTILATOR (OR ASV)

An adaptive servo-ventilator (or ASV) device is often used for people with mixed apneas (obstructive and central) or central sleep apnea. Central apneas happen when there's no physical obstruction to breathing and the brain doesn't send a signal to your diaphragm to breathe. To be eligible for this device, your ratio of central-to-obstructive events has to be more than 50%. Sometimes, central apneas can occur during CPAP titration (called treatment-emergent central apneas), especially when the pressure gets very high. This can also be an indication of the need for ASV therapy.

> **True or False? APAPs must wait for a breathing event before adjusting pressure.**
>
> In general, APAPs are programmed to act proactively, rather than reactively. Resmed's APAP devices, for example, have three different ways of detecting and preventing upper airway collapse (inspiratory flow limitation, snoring and apneas). DeVilbiss' algorithm will detect snoring and make pressure changes, since snoring usually precedes hypopneas or apneas. Other major manufacturers use similar, but proprietary, algorithms.

Bi-level, auto-bi-level and ASV devices are used as respirators in hospitals, and are sometimes called respiratory assist devices (RAD).

COMFORT FEATURES: WHAT WORKS AND WHAT DOESN'T

Although the basics of CPAP therapy haven't really changed much over the past 30 years, various comfort features have been developed that can make a significant difference.

For many new CPAP users, it's difficult to fall asleep with a mask attached to your face and with forced air blowing in. Most machines will have a ramp feature, where the pressure is gradually increased to reach your set pressure over a predefined timeframe. One problem with using this feature is that mask leaks may not show up until you've reached your optimal pressure. To solve this potential problem, another solution is to perform the mask fit test, where pressing a button can give you 10 seconds of a relatively high pressure, so you can tell instantly if your mask is experiencing a leak.

One common complaint about CPAP is that it's hard to breathe out, even at low pressures. Before moving on to a more expensive bi-level device, a new feature that tackles this problem provides a slight lowering of the pressure at the beginning of each exhalation. It's not a sudden flat lowering, as with bi-level devices, but rather a brief lowering that comes back up to the prescribed pressure very quickly. The degree of pressure relief can be manually adjusted by the user. Some trade names for this function include EPR (ResMed), and C-Flex or Bi-Flex (Philips-Respironics).

Although I've had many patients tell me that they like the expiratory pressure relief feature, one study reported no significant difference in mouth dryness or nightly hours used between straight CPAP and CPAP with pressure relief after eight weeks.

Fisher & Paykel also has a feature called SensAwake™. It detects when you wake up completely at night and instantly lowers the pressure. Not being able to fall back asleep again while using CPAP is a commonly reported problem.

With all these new 'comfort' features, it's difficult to predict whether you will be able to sleep better overall if you have any or all of these options. Some people tell me that the features do help, but others tell me that it doesn't make any difference. Everyone has different preferences, so you can't say that one manufacturer is better than another.

Size and Looks Do Matter

This next option isn't really a comfort feature, but rather a size issue. The Z1 CPAP machine from Human Design Medical is promoted to be the smallest and lightest CPAP machine, weighing only 10 oz. and measuring about 6 x 3 x 2 inches. This is without the battery pack or humidification chamber. Some of the newer models don't even look like a medical device. One model in particular (Icon+ from Fisher & Paykel) actually looks like an alarm clock.

Humidification Issues

Jason, the 55-year-old teacher, was feeling great for the first four months after starting CPAP. However, one night at 3 AM, he woke up feeling like he was drowning. After opening his eyes, he felt a gush of water coming through the mask!

Aside from the mask itself, humidification issues can either make or break your CPAP experience. Even 10 years ago, humidification was only considered an option for most patients. Doctors could prescribe either a cool water pass-over humidifier or a heated humidifier. Pass-over humidifiers work by passing air from the CPAP machine over a chamber filled with room temperature air. We now know that this design isn't strong enough to make any significant difference in terms of humidity settings. These days, heated humidification is standard, with numerous studies showing that using it can significantly increase CPAP usage and comfort levels. It's also one of the few comfort features that you can control.

In the early years of CPAP, humidification was only an option, but now it's considered essential. In fact, it is one of the most important aspects that help you to use your CPAP machine, but it's also the feature that creates so many problems or headaches. As you can imagine, regular cleaning of the water chamber can be a challenge for many people. More recent studies have shown that some people can do just as well without any humidity.

Passing dry air can cause a lot of nasal problems, including dryness, crusting, nosebleeds and nasal congestion. If your nose is congested, then you're more likely to open your mouth. This can worsen mouth leaks, which can lessen the effectiveness of CPAP. Therefore, if your nose gets congested when starting out with CPAP, one option is to try increasing your humidity level.

At the other extreme, you can have too much humidification. Depending on what type of climate you live in and how much humidity you have in your bedroom, humidity levels from CPAP machines can vary greatly. Some newer models actually adjust humidity levels based on the room's temperature and ambient humidity levels.

Another common problem with CPAP is what's called 'rain-out.' Since the air being forced through the tube is humidified, and if the air temperature in the room is cooler, water vapor inside the tube will condense, forming drops of water. This will lead to a gush of water coming out of your mask at certain times. There are a number of ways to deal with this issue (which we'll talk about in more detail in Chapter 6), but two options are to lower humidification or cover the tubing.

Manufacturers now use sophisticated algorithms and heated tubing to minimize rainout. You'll find various names attached to this technology, including ClimateLine™ (ResMed), Ambient Tracking™ (Fischer & Paykel), and ThermoSmart™ (Fisher & Paykel). Third-party CPAP supply resellers also sell simple CPAP hose covers, which may be all you need to eliminate the problem. This is what Jason experienced. It turned out that the temperature dropped in his area, but he had not turned the heat on in his house.

According to manufacturers, the water tank should be emptied and washed every day. Every manufacturer will also have slightly different recommended cleaning regimens. Since everyone will have different patterns of use, everyone will have different cleaning schedules. Emptying the tank every day and washing it once per week is probably a reasonable schedule, but your requirements may vary. Rinsing the tank with some white vinegar in water once a week is also generally recommended to disinfect the tank.

What Type of Water Should I Use for CPAP?

Manufacturers recommend using distilled water. In general, this recommendation is not for safety reasons, but more for the durability of the water chamber and the machine. Mineral deposits from tap water can build up and potentially damage the machine. If you're in a bind or if you're traveling, it's okay to use bottled water, but try to go back to using distilled water as soon as possible.

There are some reports of people successfully using boiled water or water from reverse osmosis. Regardless, if your water chamber gets covered with grimy material too quickly, then it's probably time to re-evaluate your choice of water.

Some CPAP users report adding fragrances to the water supply for aromatherapy. This is probably not a good idea, since you want to keep the water chamber as clean as possible.

Maintaining your new CPAP machine is like maintaining a new car. It needs to be taken care of and maintained on a regular basis. This is why it's so important to go through your CPAP manual and familiarize yourself with the basics of your particular make and model. Only after mastering the fundamentals should you start learning how to use the more advanced features. Focusing too early on features like end-pressure relief or arousal detection algorithms is like learning how to do a fancy jump shot before learning how to dribble the ball. Only after you learn the basics of CPAP will you be able to properly use your resources, especially if you need to troubleshoot any problems that may arise in the future.

CHAPTER 2

CPAP Masks: What Can Make or Break You

• • •

"If I find 10,000 ways something won't work, I haven't failed. I am not discouraged, because every wrong attempt discarded is another step forward."

—THOMAS EDISON

SUZY IS A 49-YEAR-OLD SCULPTOR who noticed that her sleep quality had been getting progressively worse over the past four to five years. She never felt like she slept more than two to three hours, despite getting eight hours of sleep every night. She was taking an array of anti-anxiety and high blood pressure medications, but despite all of these 'medical issues,' her sleep study showed that she only had mild sleep apnea. When she tried CPAP for the first time in the lab, she had a panic attack and ripped off her mask. Despite this negative first impression, Suzy refused to give up. After multiple visits with her sleep physician and after trying three different masks, she was able to use CPAP for longer periods of time. Three months later, she told me that she thinks she's sleeping better, because she isn't feeling as anxious as before starting CPAP.

The mask (or nasal interface) is probably the most important piece of CPAP equipment that can ultimately determine whether or not you can use your machine. The mask forms an airtight seal around your nose or around your nose and mouth, and is held in place by various types of headgear. The mask is also attached to a soft flexible hose that connects to your machine.

Notice that I said airtight, not tightly fitting. The seal must be strong enough to prevent the set air pressure from leaking, but it doesn't have to be strapped too tightly. Some of the newer masks have a soft cushioning system that inflates with air coming in from the machine, forming a proper seal. Tightening the headgear strap too much can actually cause *more* leaks.

There are three general styles of masks. The most commonly prescribed mask is the standard nasal mask, which goes over your nose. The full-face mask goes over your nose and mouth, while nasal pillows have two cushions or prongs that are placed underneath your nostrils. There are images of hundreds of different variations of these masks online if you search for CPAP masks.

Most people would probably prefer the nasal pillows at first glance, but one of the disadvantages of nasal pillows is that they can't accommodate higher pressures. You'll do fine at pressures lower than 10, but once you reach 14 or higher, you may find it more uncomfortable, due to the fact that the total pressure is delivered within a much smaller surface area. The regular nasal mask has a much larger surface area, so the average pressure that's applied to the area of the nostrils alone is much lower.

This doesn't mean that you can't try nasal pillows if your CPAP pressure is 14. Many people can use nasal pillows at higher pressure, but more people who need a higher pressure find success with a regular nasal mask.

Masks also have holes that vent out a small amount of air. This is a normal function of the mask, as it allows carbon dioxide to escape while still maintaining optimal pressure. If you can't tolerate the noise from one mask, then try switching to a different mask.

The full-face mask forms a seal over your nose and mouth. Because your mouth is also covered, this is the mask that is more likely to produce feelings of claustrophobia. It's also much bigger, bulkier, and due to the extra surface area you have to cover, higher pressure may be needed and it is much more difficult to form a good seal. There's also some concern by some sleep physicians that the mask can push on the lower jaw, moving your tongue backward, potentially creating more apneas.

The full face mask's advantage is that if you tend to breathe through your mouth, using only a nasal mask or nasal pillows will likely cause air to leak out of your mouth, lowering the optimal pressure that's needed to reach your throat. People who mouth-breathe due to having a stuffy nose sometimes complain of having a dry mouth at night. Even if you're normally a nose-breather, air leaking out your mouth can create a dry mouth. Lastly, full-face masks are the best for very high pressures. However, with higher pressure, you also have a higher chance of leaks.

There's one unusual type of mask that's worth mentioning. It's called SleepWeaver®, and it's made entirely of soft fabric, similar to the outer shell of a ski jacket. It has no latex or silicone-based materials. It's also machine washable. I have a number of patients that swear by it. However, there have also been others that didn't like it. Just like any variation of a CPAP mask, there will be some who like it and some who don't.

There are also newer variations of masks or ways of securing the mask to your nose or mouth. CPAP Pro® uses a dental mold attached to a nasal pillow system, which eliminates headgear and straps entirely. The Oracle system by Fisher & Paykel goes through only the mouth. There are also hybrid models that include nasal pillows with a full-face mask.

Most masks use three different types of materials to form a seal on your face. The first type is an air cushion-type seal, where the CPAP pressure itself is used to create a cushion of air on your face to create that suction feel. These are the masks that, if you overtighten the straps, you'll actually break the seal and create more leaks. There are also gel materials or hybrid gel and air cushions. Lastly, some masks use foam to create a cushion. All three materials work well in general, but people may prefer one over another. Everyone has different facial shapes and geometry, so one mask will not fit every face. It's also important to remember that some people may be allergic or sensitive to various materials included in the mask.

Work with your DME to ensure that you get the right size mask. Every manufacturer has mask-sizing gauges that can be printed off the Internet.

More recently, masks are being made specifically for women's smaller facial features, in more feminine colors. Various headgear and strap options are also more widely available.

The Best CPAP Mask Is the One That Works

One of the most common questions I get asked is, "What's the best mask?" My answer is usually, "The one that works best for you." Since everyone has a different face, it's hard to predict which mask will work best without trying different options. In general, most people do well with the first mask they're given, but some people have to go through three to five masks before finding one that works well.

Suzy found out about the SleepWeaver® mask through a friend, and although skeptical in the beginning, found that she could sleep much better with it.

It's also important to work with someone knowledgeable about CPAP masks to help you with the mask fitting and to troubleshoot any problems that may arise. This can happen during your follow-up visit with your sleep doctor, or with your DME provider during the initial set-up phase.

Once you find one that you like, try to have a backup available in case your current mask becomes damaged or lost.

Try Different Masks

Most CPAP mask companies have 30-day trial periods, so if you don't like a particular mask, you can try a different mask. You'll need to work with your DME company to help you with mask selection, depending on what problems you're experiencing. There are now literally hundreds of different models, sizes, and variations of masks. It's impossible to try every mask, but with the right guidance from your sleep healthcare providers or even through online forums, there's a very good possibility that you'll eventually find a mask that you like and that delivers good results.

Remember that the mask your friend likes may not fit your face very well, since everyone has a different face. There is no perfect mask. The only way to fit your face perfectly is to have a custom mask specifically made for your face. As you can imagine, this would be very expensive, and insurance probably won't pay for it.

The mask you're given in the sleep lab is usually the most basic mask. If it works, then keep using it. If not, move on to another mask. Be proactive. As with everything in life, the squeaky wheel gets the grease.

THE IMPORTANCE OF HEADGEAR, STRAPS AND OTHER COMFORT FEATURES

Much of the discussion about CPAP tends to focus on masks and machines, but there is little mention about headgear or straps. These are the components that keep the mask on your face. If it doesn't do a good job, then your mask will leak or come off during the night. Straps can come across your face from various directions, depending on the style of the mask. Sometimes the straps themselves can be irritating or annoying. As I mentioned before, some masks are designed to have straps that work without being too tight. Over-tightening can create more leaks or more discomfort. Because they run across your face, they may irritate or cause an allergic reaction. Sometimes, they can be just plain painful.

If the straps or headgear are too uncomfortable for you, the first thing you should do is talk to your equipment company. They should have the expertise to find a solution for you. Depending on what's causing the problem, and where it's happening, strap liners or covers may be recommended. One great website that sells strap covers is padacheek.com. Karen Moore, the founder of this site, has a passion for what she does, since she suffered for years from strap discomfort before discovering that a simple cover can make all the difference in the world. She also offers an assortment of mask liners that prevent skin breakdown or bruising, as well as CPAP tube covers that help to prevent rainout, which is when water condenses in the tube.

Jason, the teacher mentioned in the last chapter, started to experience some irritation on the bridge of his nose after changing to a different style mask six months after his old mask broke. He considered changing back to his old mask model, but his DME recommended that he try a mask liner. Liners are made of various types of materials, from fabric to gel-type materials. It fits between the mask and your face, lessening any chances of skin irritation or air leak.

Jason was happy that all it took was a change in liners to get back to using his CPAP regularly and thereby continuing to receive benefits from it. As Jason and so many of my other patients have told me, it's often the small issues and not necessarily the huge problems along the way that can ultimately make or break your experience with CPAP.

CHAPTER 3

Insurance Matters:
Use It or Lose It

• • •

"You snooze, you lose…"

—*Anonymous*

I ONCE RECEIVED A FRANTIC phone call from Louise, a 55-year-old woman who was upset that her insurance wanted her CPAP to be returned, since she wasn't using it long enough every night. She was using it regularly, at least four hours every night, but had skipped three nights recently when she forgot to bring it on one of her trips. Without it, she can't function.

Like Louise, many first-time CPAP users don't understand – let alone appreciate – the importance of regular CPAP use. More importantly, if your CPAP therapy is covered through your insurance company, you're not only accountable to your physician to use the CPAP regularly, but you're also accountable to your insurance company to do the same.

This section will describe CPAP data reporting and how your medical insurers use this to determine whether or not you get to hold on to your CPAP after the first few months. Moreover, you'll also learn why monitoring your own data can work to your advantage: it can be a way for you to take back control of your own health and your life.

PAP COMPLIANCE MATTERS

PAP machines are generally covered by insurance carriers. Most are paid for by the insurance company outright, so it's yours to keep, but sometimes it's on a rent-to-own plan. Medicare pays for it in increments for 13 months. On month 14, it's yours. However, beginning in 2008, Medicare implemented a three-month trial period where you have to demonstrate that you're using the machine at least four hours per night, for 70% of nights, over 30 consecutive days. You also need to meet with your sleep physician and he or she has to document that you have significant improvement in daytime sleepiness, observed apneas or morning headaches. Some insurance companies also follow Medicare's model. The only requirement is that you're able to use it for the minimum time required, and that your sleep physician attests that you are benefitting from it to a significant degree.

If you don't meet these criteria, you may lose your CPAP machine unless you see your sleep physician again, who can advocate for another 60-day extension. Again, not all insurance companies follow this model, so it's important to check with your carrier.

PAP DATA MATTERS

Most modern machines have full data reporting capabilities, including hours used, apnea-hypopnea index (AHI), average pressure, and air leaks. The AHI is the number of times you have an apnea or hypopnea every hour. Since it indirectly measures your AHI at your treatment pressure, it's almost like doing a sleep study every night. Some of the more advanced models will tell you if you have any snoring, flow limitations (partial obstructions that aren't severe enough to be called apneas or hypopneas), or even central apneas (no obstruction at all, but due to a lack of brain signals to your diaphragm).

Although the accuracy of this data is pretty good, it's not nearly as good as a formal sleep study, so you'll have to take it with a grain of salt. One statistic that's been quoted in research literature is that CPAP machine data can be off in either direction by 20%, as compared to formal sleep studies. Furthermore, each manufacturer uses different definitions of apnea and hypopneas, so you can't compare one brand to another. Ultimately, what's more important is how you feel. Some people feel great with residual apneas, whereas others won't feel any better, despite having essentially no apneas or hypopneas. The data should be used as a guide, along with various other factors such as how you feel, how well you function, and other health barometers, like your blood pressure, glucose levels, etc.

The data is typically stored on a small memory card, such as an SD card, which is a standard format for most PCs and Macs. Don't worry if you have to remove your card. A copy of the data is stored in the machine. Most of the newer models will give you a summary of your night's sleep on the display screen, so you don't have to check the card or computer every morning.

With these new powerful tools, you have the ability to take control of your own care. However, with this ability also comes additional responsibility. Ideally, you can check your data every few weeks or months on a regular basis to see how you're doing, and make the necessary adjustments.

In the old days, you had to drop off or mail in your card to your sleep physician, who would then extract and interpret the data. Depending on the results, an order might be placed by your sleep doctor to make any pressure changes with the DME, who would either come to your house to make the changes, or have you go back to the sleep lab to make the changes. In other cases, the card would be sent to the equipment company, who would then send the information to your sleep physician, who would send an order back to the equipment company to make any adjustments. The card would be mailed back with the new machine settings. Obviously, this is a very long and convoluted process.

Years ago, for some odd reason, sleep doctors were reluctant to give patients direct access to their own data. The software required to read the data was difficult to get, and you had to go through hoops to install it on your computer once you gained access. The good news is that sleep doctors' opinions are changing, and the entire industry is generally headed toward more open and easier access for patients to read their own data. There's even a free open-source program (SleepyHead) that can read most of the popular CPAP models. Each of the major manufacturers also has better options, and they are now beginning to integrate online web services where you can upload the data from your computer. Philips Respironics has an app called DreamMapper. ResMed has myAir. New apps and programs for other manufacturers are constantly being developed.

Nowadays, CPAP machines can also be configured to connect to your home Wi-Fi network, allowing your physician or DME to look at your data in real time, and even make pressure adjustments remotely.

I can envision a time when you'll be connected automatically to your computer and it will send you periodic progress reports, or alert you if there's a problem or something to look into. Your physicians and DME can also be alerted when this happens and subsequently take appropriate action.

PAP Insurance Issues

Since PAP devices are categorized as DME (durable medical goods) equipment, any copays, coinsurance or deductibles will apply. Most insurance will cover CPAP for sleep apnea. Medicare usually pays 80% of what's allowed. The remainder is either your responsibility or your supplemental insurance may pick it up. In rare cases, some patients won't have DME coverage. Your sleep lab or DME can find out this information for you, or you can talk to your health benefits contact person.

All the different supplies (PAP, humidifier, mask, tubing, headgear, etc.) are billed separately. This is why you'll see so many items on your insurance carrier's explanation of benefits.

For the disposable parts, most insurance companies are on a three to six-month schedule. Medicare is on a three-month cycle. Your DME can tell you what your schedule is. Replacement parts for the mask (nasal pillow cushions, straps, etc.) can be replaced at any time if they break. It's a good idea to put this date on your calendar beforehand so you don't forget and have to scramble to replace a broken mask. If you have a backup mask on hand, it can save you from aggravation in the future if your current mask breaks.

Remember that all CPAP equipment and related supplies require a prescription from your physician.

What If You Don't Have Insurance?

Worst-case scenario, if you don't have insurance, you can purchase equipment through a DME or an online CPAP store. You'll need a prescription to do this. I've seen basic new CPAP machines sold for as low as $200. APAP and bi-level machines will cost more. The mask will range anywhere from $100 to $200. You also have to take into consideration the additional equipment and supplies, such as humidification, headgear, tubing, etc. A basic middle-of-the-road system with all the accessories you'll need will cost somewhere between $500 and $1000.

If you're in dire financial straits, the American Sleep Apnea Association (ASAA) does have a CPAP Assistance Program. If you have a PAP machine that you're not using, please consider donating it to the ASAA. SecondwindCPAP.com is a place where you can also sell and buy used CPAP equipment. If you use these online sites, it's still important to work with your sleep physician to make sure that you're being treated appropriately.

The PAP machine is an air blower, so nothing can contaminate it internally (except for the water you use), but I strongly recommend that you order a new mask, headgear and tubing.

Fortunately for Louise, her 'lack of compliance' didn't end up costing her the CPAP machine that she needed so badly. She called to make an appointment to see me quickly and I extended her CPAP trial period. She was able to use the CPAP machine for seven to eight hours nightly for 30 consecutive days, and was thrilled to hold on to her CPAP machine.

Summary

John Wooden's quote at the beginning of Chapter 1 emphasizes the details and mastering the fundamentals whenever you want to succeed in an endeavor. He also points out that the most successful people have failed many times before becoming successful. Some of the most famous examples of this include Sam Walton, Henry Ford, and Abraham Lincoln.

The fundamentals not only include having a basic understanding of how CPAP works, routine maintenance and troubleshooting, but also about insurance requirements and financial considerations.

Now that you understand the basic fundamentals of CPAP, you're ready to deal with some important mindset issues about CPAP, as well as other important troubleshooting steps, which I'll cover in the next few chapters.

Mindset and CPAP Troubleshooting

• • •

"The mind is a powerful thing. It can take you through walls."

—DENIS AVEY
AUTHOR, *THE MAN WHO BROKE INTO AUSCHWITZ:
A TRUE STORY OF WORLD WAR II*

CHAPTER 4

The One Solution for All Your CPAP Problems

• • •

"We cannot solve our problems with the same thinking we used when we created them."

—ALBERT EINSTEIN

JONATHAN IS A COLLEGE SENIOR in his early 20s who was newly diagnosed with obstructive sleep apnea. He was very physically active in college. I explained to him all his different treatment options and then recommended CPAP, expecting him to refuse. Surprisingly, he was more than willing to try CPAP. It turns out that his best friend has sleep apnea and has been happy using CPAP.

When it comes to accepting and using CPAP, the biggest barrier to overcome is not how cumbersome CPAP is, or even how adaptable you can be to new forms of therapy. **It's your mindset**. What I've learned from seeing thousands of OSA patients succeed and fail with CPAP therapy is that it's your prior knowledge of various options, what your friends and family have told you, or previous experiences that affect you the most. These are the things that influence whether or not you'll begin using CPAP, and whether or not you continue using it despite various problems that may arise.

For many people with newly diagnosed obstructive sleep apnea, the thought of having to use a mask every night can be disturbing. Over the past 15 years, I've heard almost every possible objection to CPAP whenever I recommend it as an option. In general, there are two types of people when CPAP is first introduced: the ones that gladly accept CPAP and are enthusiastic about using it, and those that are reluctant from the start. Unfortunately, for many of my patients, it's often their mindset and not necessarily their ability to use it or the severity of their sleep apnea condition that determines whether or not they'll be successful. I say unfortunately because those who have negative preconceptions about CPAP are doomed even before they start. Fortunately, for the majority of you, this is good news, because your mindset is something you can change.

Carol Dweck, noted author of *Mindset: The New Psychology of Success*, points out that people can have either fixed or growth mindsets. People who eventually succeed are willing to take on fears and challenges and see them as opportunities to grow and learn. People with fixed mindsets are those who won't even consider trying CPAP, despite all the potential benefits.

If you're ready and willing to give CPAP a try, you can skip this chapter altogether. However, it may be worthwhile to learn about common objections that people have about CPAP so that you can help others who may have these issues.

THE SEVEN STAGES OF CPAP

Being diagnosed with obstructive sleep apnea and using CPAP for the first time can be traumatic, like the death of a loved one, a divorce, or a major job change. It's a major life change, and there are common stages that everyone undergoes. Mike Moran posted a very insightful essay on CPAPtalk.com that I summarize here, called The Seven Stages of CPAP:

1. **Denial**. This is a common trait with many sleep apnea sufferers. The last thing you want to admit is that you snore like a train. Snoring is something everyone laughs about and you don't want the embarrassment of being the brunt of a joke.

2. **Realization**. Your spouse tells you that you are constantly gasping and choking at night, and after doing some research, you finally realize why you're so cranky and tired during the day. Learning about the dangers of untreated obstructive sleep apnea is an eye-opening experience.

3. **Diagnosis**. A formal overnight sleep study confirms that you stop breathing over 50 times every hour, with your oxygen levels dropping to levels below 80%. A CPAP study confirms that your apneas are completely controlled at the measured setting.

4. **Frustration**. This can start from the time you undergo the sleep study, or are waiting for the CPAP machine to arrive, and even after you start using your CPAP machine. It's like waiting for a biopsy result after a breast or colon biopsy to make sure it's not cancer. You'll experience a combination of anticipation, due to possibly sleeping better for the first time in years, as well as the fear and anxiety of possibly having to use a machine on your face for the rest of your life. There can be a delay in your CPAP machine delivery, which only aggravates your frustrations. Once you start using your machine, you might not get the relief that you're expecting. There are a number of major and minor issues that you relay to your sleep doctors and your equipment company, but it's been difficult to get an answer from anyone.

5. **Immersion**. You work tirelessly with your doctors and equipment providers, bugging them to the point of possibly being annoying.

You scour the Internet and connect with other like-minded CPAP users, devouring as much information as possible to accomplish your mission: to get better sleep. You test various different masks or machines, different gadgets, and other options that make your CPAP use more beneficial.

6. **Ownership**. You take responsibility for your own care, and you don't have to depend on your doctors or equipment providers. You still work with your healthcare providers, but you take the initiative to ask the right questions and modify your treatment regimen to see what works or doesn't work.

7. **Inflation**. You may get only a few hours of sleep in the beginning, but the periods are now getting longer and longer. You don't wake up to a "Wow" morning, but you're beginning to realize that you're not as tired in the late afternoon as you used to be, or you're not falling asleep in certain situations. The progress in this stage can fluctuate over time, but becomes more consistent as time passes.

The 10 Most Common CPAP Objections

It's only human nature to want to avoid sleeping strapped to a mask potentially for the rest of your life. Many people are able to go through the seven stages of CPAP use with some or significant benefits. But for those that are still struggling, here are the ten most common objections that I hear from patients, along with my responses:

1. I can't imagine wearing that contraption strapped to my face every night. I know that I won't use it.

This is one of the most common objections I get whenever I recommend CPAP. It's only natural. You already have problems sleeping. It doesn't seem like the kind of thing anyone would willingly do, no matter what the benefit may be. Sleep is supposed to be about relaxation, comfort and ease, but seeing those CPAP contraptions for the first time can conjure up the complete opposite feeling in anyone. And no wonder, since more often than not, the closest thing they've seen that resembles anything like it is usually worn by deathly ill people in intensive care units. For many of us, even thinking about sleeping with a mask attached to a hose can create feelings of anxiety, panic or even horror.

However, despite these negative first impressions, it's surprising how often people who go through with a CPAP study tell me it wasn't that bad. This doesn't necessarily equate to sleeping much better, but the simple act of sleeping with CPAP wasn't as bad as what they expected. This fear is similar to various phobias or anxieties that people suffer from, such as a fear of heights or open spaces. It's a type of fear that's exaggerated in the mind even before giving it a try.

Some of you may shudder at the thought of using a mask attached to a machine for the rest of your life. Chip Smith of Restoration Medical Supply suggests thinking about CPAP as a 'fountain of youth.' Using CPAP effectively can definitely slow down or prevent premature aging or death.

2. I'M CLAUSTROPHOBIC.

For people with claustrophobia (fear of closed or small spaces), the thought of using a mask that covers your nose or mouth can cause a mini panic attack. If you're one of these people, it's likely that you'll refuse to try it altogether. This is unfortunate, since there are a number of desensitization techniques that are available for CPAP, similar to those used for people with claustrophobia. Dweck, the author of *Mindset, The New Psychology of Success*, argues that the fear of the unknown often derails us, rather than the experience itself. Oftentimes, simply improving nasal breathing can also make a huge difference.

3. It's not sexy. I don't want to look like Darth Vader. Having something strapped to your face can seem like a deterrent to romantic situations.

Being exhausted and sleep deprived from years of untreated obstructive sleep apnea can significantly lower your sex drive and intimacy levels. Obstructive sleep apnea has also been shown to reduce sex hormone levels and cause fertility problems. Putting on the mask on a regular basis after you're finished making love doesn't seem like such a bad trade off after all.

4. I travel a lot.

As more and more of our economy shifts from domestic to global, it's inevitable that more and more of my patients, both young and old, will fly frequently. In many situations, traveling anywhere from two to three days in a week for work has become the norm for my patients. CPAP no longer operates under the assumption that 'one size fits all,' despite what many of the early adopters and the media often portray.

CPAP machines come in a dizzying array of sizes, making them more portable than ever. Most can fit comfortably inside a small backpack, along with all the required accessories. One particular model (Human Design Medical's Z1) weighs less than one pound and measures about 6 x 3 x 2 inches. CPAP can also be used on long flights (seats with power), and can even be used in areas without power (using battery packs).

Therefore, the question you need to ask yourself is—if you are willing to carry around your laptop computer, iPad, iPhone and a cornucopia of electronic gadgets on the plane to ease your travel for work or play, and for a mere one pound extra you can take along the ultimate gadget that can help you do all of those things more efficiently and effectively, since you'll be able to get the sleep you need to live the life you want—why wouldn't you want to do this?

5. MY FATHER USED **CPAP**—I DON'T WANT TO DO WHAT HE DID.

This is a common objection. Seeing your parent use a machine every night can create feelings of curiosity or fear. The fact that your mother or father had obstructive sleep apnea is very relevant, since you inherited your anatomy from your parents. Oftentimes, younger patients with OSA miss the fact that they will probably inherit their parents' other medical conditions as well. A common statement by such a patient is, "My father has high blood pressure and had a heart attack when he was in his 60s. I'm healthy now." When I point out that untreated obstructive sleep apnea can cause high blood pressure and significantly raise your risk of a heart attack later in life, most people quickly change their minds.

6. I CAN'T BREATHE THROUGH MY NOSE.

This is an easily treatable problem using anything from saline irrigation or nasal dilator devices to medications or surgery. In fact, studies have shown that improving nasal breathing, in general, can improve CPAP tolerance and usage.

7. I CAN'T AFFORD IT, OR I DON'T HAVE INSURANCE.

Medical equipment can be expensive, especially if you go through standard list prices that are given to insurance companies. However, online prices can be much more reasonable, with some basic models in the $300 to $500 range. You can even find secondhand, refurbished CPAP machines for around $200 to $300. I just saw a listing for a new CPAP machine on sale for under $200. Also, the American Sleep Apnea Association has its CPAP assistance program. The one advantage to going through a durable medical equipment company is that they will give you customized, in-person assistance, as opposed to virtual or online support.

8. IT'S TOO NOISY. MY WIFE CAN'T SLEEP WITH ANY NOISE.

Modern CPAP machines are very quiet. Every model is different, but most people describe the noise as being like a soft whisper. Most models have sound levels in the 25 to 30 dB range, which is much more preferable to the loud snoring one will hear in the absence of CPAP, which can reach levels of up to 90 dB (the level of a motorcycle at 25 feet).

9. I CAN'T REMEMBER TO PUT ON A MASK EVERY NIGHT.

If you often fall asleep watching TV, or get home at odd hours every night, then remembering to put on the CPAP may be impractical, if not impossible. Ultimately, whether or not you develop this important habit will depend on how important sleep is for you. If it's important, you'll find ways of remembering every night. Some patients, who are willing to make this work, even begin wearing the mask one to two hours before they retire to bed. This helps them not only to remember to hook it up to the machine before they go to sleep, but once acclimated, they're less likely to have the negative associations they may have had about wearing a mask while they try to fall sleep.

10. I DON'T LIKE ANYTHING ON MY FACE.

Some people are very sensitive to anything on their face or bodies, or they are extremely light sleepers. Until you try it, you don't know what you'll like or dislike. I often like to challenge my young children to try new foods or learn new skills by asking them, "What's the worst thing that can happen?" In the same way, I ask these patients to recall specific moments in their lives when they've tried something that they thought they'd hate, but to their surprise, they ended up liking it once they tried it. Trying something new, especially if it entails a long commitment and seems to pose a threat to our comfort level, is a valid objection that many of us have.

Even I will admit that I don't like trying new things. However, in many cases with CPAP users, OSA is not something that will go away. Unlike your initial discomfort from the mask, which will eventually dissipate the more you use it, the worst that can happen if you don't treat severe sleep apnea is that you'll shorten your lifespan.

Notice that all these fears and objections are brought up before patients even try CPAP. No matter how reluctant you may be about using CPAP, you won't know how it feels unless you try it. Granted, it's possible that you may tell me, "See, I told you so." However, there are many people who tell me afterwards, "Surprisingly, I slept great!" Another comment was, "I only slept two hours, but I slept really well." Worst-case scenario—if you still hate it, you can check it off the list and move on to other options, such as dental devices or surgery.

Starting with CPAP is not expected to give you a great night's sleep on the very first night. This does happen occasionally, but for most people, it's a process that can take weeks or even months before they begin to sleep better. Albert Einstein once said that insanity is doing the same thing over and over again and expecting different results. Without constant trouble-shooting and vigilance in terms of how effectively you sleep using CPAP, you'll never be able to improve your sleep quality.

Summary

Jonathan was fortunate that he had a positive experience with a close friend who loved sleeping with his CPAP. While some people start sleeping great from their very first night using CPAP, the vast majority of users will go through the seven phases described above at different speeds. It's important to do your research and communicate with your doctors to troubleshoot whatever problem you may encounter, and be constantly checking your progress, even if you've reached the point where you're happy. Something will always be changing, whether it's your CPAP pressure needs, your weight, weather changes, or even your quality of nasal breathing, which can affect how well CPAP works for you.

CHAPTER 5

CPAP Stickiness: What Research Shows Versus What Users Say

• • •

"It does not matter how slowly you go as long as you do not stop."

—*Confucius*

KEITH IS A 59-YEAR-OLD BUS driver for New York City Transit who came to see me about what he suspected to be sleep apnea, based on his slowly increasing fatigue and frequent memory lapses. When he was diagnosed with moderate sleep apnea, he was relieved to find out that he would be able to keep his job, as long as he was able to use CPAP on a regular basis and get cleared by his sleep doctor. He gave it his best shot, but after 30 days, Keith was not able to use his CPAP for more than two to three hours per night. Not being able to meet the requirements of being 'adherent,' his CPAP was taken away.

Now he's angry because his proactive effort to take care of his sleep apnea problem didn't produce the positive outcome he expected. From his perspective, he did all the right things, for the right reasons, and got punished for the effort. I often see many unhappy sleep apnea sufferers experience this as a result of seemingly arbitrary guidelines set by the government and sleep doctors.

Whenever sleep doctors talk about CPAP effectiveness, we use words like compliance and adherence. I like the word stickiness, since it is a good description for how attached you are to your CPAP machine. It doesn't, however, mean how greasy or grimy your machine is after years of neglect!

Essentially, as I mentioned earlier in Chapter 3, when I talked about how insurance carriers determine their CPAP eligibility and coverage, the number of hours you use your CPAP on a nightly basis is what's measured. The older term for this was compliance, which means cooperation or yielding to recommendations for CPAP use. These days, we use the term adherence, which means sticking to or holding fast to CPAP use. The gold standard definition of adherence set forth by Medicare is defined as greater than four hours of use per night on 70% of nights, during a consecutive 30-day period, at any time during the first three months of initial usage.

This is also what most insurance companies use to decide whether or not you get to hold on to your CPAP machine. Notice, if you normally sleep eight hours per night, using this criteria you'll have to use CPAP for only 35% of total sleep time over one month to meet these criteria. If you normally sleep seven hours per night, this figure is 40%. The other criterion to determine if you get to hold on to your CPAP machine is that the treating physician has to document that sleep symptoms have improved within the second or third month of treatment.

The beauty of newer CPAP machines is that they will tell you exactly how many hours each night you use your machine. In addition, some can also tell you if you still stop breathing, along with reporting mask air leak rates. Some advanced machines can even tell you if you have central apneas while on CPAP therapy.

So why is this important? Numerous studies have shown that using CPAP effectively for at least four hours per night lowers sleepiness, improves daily functioning and restores memory to normal levels.[1] The powers that be (Medicare and the sleep physicians) had to set a bare minimum threshold for hours used to say that CPAP makes any significant difference. As you can see, 35 to 40% of total sleep time is considered the bare minimum number of hours when using CPAP on a consistent basis to measure any significantly improved health outcomes (such as not dying early). Ideally, you should be using CPAP much more often than the bare minimum.

It's one thing to say you're able to use CPAP for four hours per night, but it's a very different thing to say that you're using it effectively during those four hours. If the machine's pressure is not set to optimal levels, or if there's a leak around the mask, the CPAP's effectiveness will be much lower, despite the fact that you're 'adherent.' Some people are 100% 'adherent,' with perfect numbers reported from the CPAP machine, but they will feel no better and might even feel worse. As you can see, we have a lot more to do in terms of raising the bar in not only getting people to use CPAP for longer periods, but also in being able to obtain meaningful measurements of sleep quality improvement.

Another issue to consider is that if you normally sleep eight hours per night, but use CPAP 'effectively' for four hours per night, your average nightly AHI will be about 50% of your original score. For example, if you start off with an AHI of 50, and use CPAP for four hours per night on average (AHI is 0 on CPAP), then your average AHI every night will be 25.

Even if Keith the bus driver had been able to use his CPAP for four hours every night successfully, he would still have untreated severe obstructive sleep apnea for the remaining four hours. To 'clear' Keith to drive a bus again, I had to certify that Keith was significantly improved and would be okay to go back to work.

Why CPAP Adherence Doesn't Equal CPAP Success

With optimal education and support, the vast majority of people can be considered CPAP 'adherent.' However, the reported non-adherence rate that has been reported in the research literature ranges from 46 to 86%.[2] It's important to note that different studies use different definitions of adherence, along with different follow-up periods, so you have to take these numbers with a grain of salt. Also, it's a well-known fact that people in research studies tend to have better results, especially if they're being followed regularly. If you spend some time researching CPAP adherence or compliance, you'll see that many of the studies report widely varying and often conflicting results.

Regardless, there are a few basic principles that are worth considering. In my personal experience, long-term adherence is much less than 50%. Here's one general rule of thumb that was summarized to me by Dr. Carl Stepnowski: Out of 100 people given CPAP, about 80% will agree to begin using CPAP. About half of those that started using CPAP will continue for at least one year, and of those people, half will be using it more than half the night. In other words, only 20 out of 100 people will be using CPAP at acceptable levels at the one-year mark.[3]

As expected, numerous studies have shown that CPAP use in the first month correlates highly with adherence six to twelve months later.[4] Compared to various other chronic health conditions that require adhering to a program or using equipment, CPAP use by people with sleep apnea is usually among the worst in terms of adherence rates.

Intensive patient education (especially in the first month) with follow-up visits and support significantly increases the chances of CPAP adherence and nightly usage. Even with intensive methods, the rate at which you will get used to CPAP therapy and use it on a regular basis is highly variable. Some people do well after only a few days. For others, it might take years.

Some even do well initially for a few months, and then struggle for a few months.

Interestingly, many of the studies that report very high adherence rates are not from the United States. A Canadian study reported 84% adherence rate at six months using a greater than four hours per night threshold.[5] A French study reported 90% usage rate at the three-year mark,[6] and a Spanish study reported that almost 80% of women are still using CPAP after 10 years.[7]

It's surprising the disconnect that I see with CPAP adherence in the US versus what I read about from other countries. What I see in clinical practice is more in line with what Dr. Stepnowski described. In countries with more centralized healthcare systems, where few options are available besides CPAP, it's likely that more people will be accepting of CPAP.

Unfortunately for those of us in the United States, CPAP compliance relies on the end user to figure out what's right and what's not, from the many conflicting opinions from doctors, surgeons, research studies and lay opinions. Then, the same user is given the awesome burden of making a choice with little or no coaching or counseling. Sometimes, having too much of a good thing (or having too many treatment options) is not such a good thing after all. Just based on the statistics alone, it seems like you're doomed to fail—or are you? There is a solution, but you must be willing to look for it… just not in the places you were expecting.

How to Succeed with CPAP Once and for All

Different people will have different preferences for the type of CPAP masks they choose, but so far, there's no evidence to say that nasal pillows or full-face masks are any better than traditional nasal masks. Age, sex, marital status, and socioeconomic status have not been consistently associated with CPAP adherence.

There's a general consensus within the sleep community that people with severe sleep apnea (AHI > 30) or severe drops in oxygen levels may be able to tolerate CPAP better than those with mild sleep apnea,[8] but other studies have not supported this. However, CPAP adherence was strongly associated with self-reported sleepiness scores. Having an Epworth sleepiness score > 10 (see Figure 1) was associated with long-term CPAP use.[9] CPAP use was low in patients with severe sleep apnea and low sleepiness scores.

Epworth Sleepiness Scale

How likely are you to doze off or fall asleep in the following situations, in contrast to just feeling tired? This questionnaire refers to your chance of falling asleep, according to your usual way of life, for about the last week or two. Even if you have not done some of these things recently, try to estimate how they would have affected you during the last two weeks.

Use the following scale to choose the most appropriate number for each situation.

0 = No chance of dozing
1 = Slight chance of dozing
2 = Moderate chance of dozing
3 = High chance of dozing

Situation:

Sitting and reading _____

Watching TV _____

Sitting inactive in a public place _____

As a passenger in a car for one hour without a break _____

Lying down to rest in the afternoon when circumstances permit _____

Sitting and talking to someone _____

Sitting quietly after lunch without alcohol _____

In a car, while stopped in traffic for a few minutes _____

Total: _____

Figure 1. Adapted from Johns, Murray W. "Daytime sleepiness, snoring, and obstructive sleep apnea: the Epworth Sleepiness Scale." Chest 103.1 (1993): 30-36.

NASAL CONGESTION

Nasal congestion is another factor that is strongly associated with lower levels of CPAP use. One recent study found that average CPAP use went from 30 minutes to over five hours every night after nasal surgery.[10] Although nasal surgery doesn't get rid of sleep apnea in most cases, patients generally feel much better subjectively, can use CPAP for longer periods, and CPAP pressures can often be lowered. This is why I'm relatively aggressive in treating nasal congestion medically or surgically before recommending CPAP for my patients. See Chapter 8 for more ways to deal with your stuffy nose.

Again, it's important to note that nasal surgery generally doesn't improve obstructive sleep apnea to a significant degree.

OTHER FACTORS

Some studies have looked at CPAP adherence between the standard two-night protocol (one night to diagnose sleep apnea and then another night to measure the right CPAP pressure), a split-night study (when the diagnostic and CPAP pressure study is done in a single night), and an unattended home titration study (an automatic PAP machine study done at home). There was no difference between the two-night vs. split-night protocols. However, a technician-attended in-lab titration study resulted in one hour more of CPAP use, as compared to the home titration study. This just goes to show that immediate feedback, troubleshooting and reinforcement are important when it comes to initial CPAP acceptance.

Psychological factors, such as having anxiety or depression, were not found to predict CPAP adherence, but patients' perception of the benefits of symptoms following CPAP use has been shown to be related to better adherence. As expected, patients who experienced greater improvements in symptoms had better adherence. Social support factors, such as having active partner participation or support group involvement, were also found to be helpful.

Nationally, CPAP adherence rates can be lower than 50%. Some DMEs can reach rates well over 80%, but this is unusual. To improve CPAP adherence, there are three general categories that are important to discuss: educational support, clinical support (mechanical issues, desensitization issues, etc.), and psychological/behavioral support. In general, the more often you see your doctor or interact with your DME, the more likely you'll continue to use CPAP. If you're still struggling with CPAP, despite frequent interactions, seeing a behavioral sleep psychologist for CPAP desensitization and cognitive behavioral therapy can be helpful.

In general, intensive CPAP intervention programs increase CPAP use by about one hour per night. One of the downsides of intensive support is that it takes much more time and human resources for your provider to make the phone calls, see patients, and visit patients in the home settings. Another way of providing intensively structured support while using fewer healthcare resources is a web-based model, where patients are educated on sleep apnea and CPAP, and receive immediate feedback on their uploaded data, with numerous support and troubleshooting options. Many CPAP manufacturers (such as Respironics and ResMed) have websites where patients can upload their CPAP data and receive immediate feedback. One extra hour of CPAP use may not seem like much, but on a long-term basis, it can make a significant difference to your overall future state of health.

Is CPAP Appropriate for Mild OSA?

While CPAP is clearly recommended for people with moderate to severe OSA, the data is still not as convincing for its use in people with mild OSA. Studies have shown that people with mild sleep apnea have significantly lower adherence rates, as compared with people suffering from moderate to severe OSA. Additionally, the higher risk factors for heart disease, heart attack and stroke were shown in studies to apply to people with moderate to severe sleep apnea.

However, there are many people who have very mild (AHI 5 to 15) or no sleep apnea (AHI < 5), but still stop breathing 20 to 30 times every hour. Because these pauses last less than 10 seconds, they are not counted as apneas or hypopneas. This is a condition called upper airway resistance syndrome, or UARS. Typically, these patients are younger and thinner, with blood pressure on the normal or low side. They will not have high blood pressure, diabetes or heart disease. Instead, they will most likely suffer from various symptoms such as chronic fatigue, headaches, anxiety or depression, insomnia, cold hands or feet, digestive problems or hypo-thyroidism. For more information about UARS, please read the article on my blog at doctorstevenpark.com. I have a much more in-depth explana-tion of why UARS occurs and how it's different from OSA in my book, *Sleep Interrupted.*

So if you only have mild obstructive sleep apnea, does it justify the time, expense, and resources required for people with lower risk factors and who are less likely to tolerate CPAP? This is an ongoing debate in the sleep medicine community. In my experience, it's hit or miss; some people feel better, but most don't. You don't know whether or not it's going to work until you try it.

Keith, the bus driver, absolutely refused to use CPAP again. However, he never refused to believe that his inability to use CPAP was going to cost him his health, let alone his job. As a result, after improving his nasal breathing with allergy medications on my recommendation, he eventually saw a dentist for a mandibular advancement device. After three adjust-ments to move his jaw forward, he began to sleep much better. His day-time fatigue also improved significantly, with his Epworth score dropping from 15 to 8. A home sleep study with his appliance showed that his sleep apnea had dropped into the mild range. Although Keith's prospects for returning to work didn't look very good during his suspension, he kept persisting until he found something that worked for him. I'm happy to say that when Keith was finally cleared to go back to work, he was all the more wiser and happier, having learned how to take control of his health, not to mention, his life.

CHAPTER 6

Your Top 15 CPAP Problems, Solved

• • •

"Start by doing what's necessary; then do what's possible;
and suddenly you are doing the impossible."

—St. Francis of Assisi

JASON, THE SCHOOL TEACHER I introduced you to in Chapter 1, did well for six months after starting CPAP, but came back to see me because he kept waking up at night to find that his mask had moved off his face. It turned out that he had changed apartments a few weeks ago, and had to change the position of his CPAP machine from above his head to the right side of his bed. It sounded like as he was turning in bed, his hose became tethered on his bed or sheets, tugging on the mask and creating air leaks. This lowered his CPAP pressure, which increased the chances that he would have an apnea more often.

A change like the one that Jason experienced makes using CPAP all the more difficult. However, the better prepared you are when the change happens, the better chance you'll have of adapting quickly.

Over the more than five years that I answered questions for my *Ask Dr. Park Teleseminars* and *Expert Interviews*, I received thousands of questions about CPAP. Unsurprisingly, the same types of questions were asked over and over. These are the top 15 that I saw most often. Reading through them will definitely help to better prepare you for many of the challenges that you'll likely encounter along the way. There are many others that I can't answer within the space limits of this book, but I do address a number of other issues in the next chapter.

PROBLEM #1: DRY MOUTH

Waking up with a dry mouth while using CPAP is a common problem. With a regular nasal mask or nasal pillows, air leaking out the mouth can cause extreme dryness, as well as lowering the necessary pressure that's needed to keep your airway open.

Solution: For regular nasal mask or nasal pillow users with mouth leaks, your two options are to try adding a chinstrap to keep your mouth closed or switch to a full-face mask. Even with full-face masks, your mouth can dry out through air convection. For this particular situation, the first thing to consider is raising the humidity level. There's usually a button on your CPAP machine to change the humidity settings.

PROBLEM #2: MY MASK IS LEAKING

If your mask leaks, you'll usually know it. Air can rush out of the side of the mask, sometimes even going into your eye. Sometimes it will make a squeaking noise that bothers your partner in bed. Even if you don't notice any leaks, your sleep quality may be suffering due to silent leaks throughout the night.

Solution: The first thing to do with any mask leak is to readjust your straps or headgear. Make sure that you have a properly fitting mask that's the right size. You may need to contact your DME provider to go over your mask fit. Remember that for some masks, tightening the straps too much can make the leaks much worse. Also remember that leaks can happen in areas away from your mask, so it's important to check the entire circuit from your mask to your machine.

Occasionally, mask leaks can happen that are not too significant, and if you're sleeping well, there's no need to do anything. Men with facial hair may need to consider shaving certain areas of their face if other mask options don't work. Facial hair issues are discussed in more detail in the next chapter.

Problem #3: CPAP is Too Noisy

Most modern CPAP machines are actually very quiet. Sound levels range from 20 to 30 dB, which is about the loudness of a soft whisper.

Solution: If your machine is making too much noise, then check for leaks throughout the entire system, from the machine to the mask. The machine may be defective, especially if it suddenly begins making a new noise. Some masks have an air release hole that produces a soft puff of air, which is normal. If this bothers you or your partner, then you can always try a different mask. Worst-case scenario, ear plugs can also be used.

People have suggested placing the machine on the floor rather than on the nightstand, but this is probably not wise since there's more dust on the ground. Another suggestion is to place a soft mat under the machine to dampen the motor's vibrations. Some people even make or purchase boxes or containers to lower sound levels.

Problem #4: The Mask Keeps Coming Off

You probably placed your CPAP machine on the nightstand next to your bed. With this configuration, it's likely that as you turn onto your other side, the tubing will become tethered and pull on your mask, causing a leak or coming off entirely. Placing the CPAP machine at the top of your head is unfortunately not an option for most people.

Solution: One of the simplest ways to help solve this problem is to route the tube to hang down from above your head. There are various hose holders that you can purchase online for a relatively low cost. Essentially, the hose is suspended above your head, rather than from one side. A simple, low-tech option that's described by Bruce Stein in his book *Sleep Apnea & CPAP* is as follows: Suspend your tubing above your head using long rubber bands. It can hang from a hook on the wall, the corners of the headboard, picture frames, or even lighting hardware. You may have to create a horizontal crossing string or wire to hang your rubber band off the middle portion. The elastic properties of the rubber band will allow the tubing to move more freely.

Jason implemented this recommendation at home, and called me back in two weeks to say that it worked, and that he is sleeping better again.

Problem #5: I'm Allergic to the Mask

Although uncommon, some people can react to CPAP mask materials, especially latex or silicone. The softer mask components that touch your face or nostrils are usually made of silicone, while the harder clear plastic base material is made of polycarbonate. Latex is now rarely used in CPAP masks, but silicone can sometimes lead to contact allergic dermatitis.

Solution: A simple solution to this is to use one of the many mask liners that are available online. Make sure that you find the right size for your particular mask. The mask straps contain neoprene, which can also cause facial or scalp irritation. The tubing is made of plastic, with most product descriptions stating that it's made of high-quality, long-lasting materials. What this means is that it's made of polyester with silicone cuffs. There's also been some concern about the presence of bisphenol-A (BPA) in CPAP materials with polycarbonate, but manufacturers claim that the levels of BPA are safe and that they meet all biomedical regulatory requirements.[1]

Problem #6: Chest Soreness After CPAP

CPAP pressure, especially if it is on the higher side, can over-inflate the lungs, causing stretching of the lining of the lungs. This can cause chest soreness or diffuse chest pain, especially when you take a deep breath.

Solution: In most cases, this slowly resolves over days or weeks, but if it doesn't, one recommendation is to sleep on your side. If this doesn't work, lowering the pressure or switching to a bi-level device are two other options. This is a decision you and your sleep doctor have to talk about.

Problem #7: Claustrophobia

Claustrophobia is a common condition that is only made worse when using a CPAP mask.

Solution: Slow acclimation is key, with incremental periods of wearing the mask without being attached to the machine (and without tubing). Nasal congestion can also aggravate feelings of claustrophobia, so this should be addressed as well. If these options don't work, you might consider seeing a behavioral sleep specialist who specializes in CPAP desensitization and cognitive behavioral therapy for insomnia and sleep problems.

Problem #8: Sinus and Ear Pain

Since your ears and nasal sinuses connect to your nose, adding pressure can sometimes push air into these cavities. Typically, with routine swallowing and normal ear and sinus functioning, built-up pressure gradually releases, but if you have any degree of inflammation (due to allergies, colds, or even from weather changes), there will be a partial blockage, so air can't escape as easily.

Solution: Temporary over-the-counter decongestants may help, but if it persists, see an ear, nose and throat (ENT) doctor for additional help. Sometimes, switching from a nasal mask to a full-face mask can help, since some of the pressure is diverted away from the sinuses and ears.

Problem #9: Stomach Bloating with CPAP Use

Sometimes, air from the CPAP machine can travel into your stomach.

Solution: The first reaction is to lower your pressure, but that will likely lower the effectiveness of your treatment. Changing your sleep position can also help. Side sleeping has also been found to improve this condition.

A recent presentation at our national sleep meeting reported the resolution of bloating in all 20 of their study patients by adding a chinstrap, applying end-pressure relief, or switching to a bi-level PAP machine.[2] The author concluded that having an air leak through the mouth could aggravate the swallowing of air. Eight out of 20 responded by using a chinstrap alone, three responded by adding end-pressure relief, and nine responded by switching to a bi-level machine.

Sometimes, bloating with CPAP can be associated with higher rates of reflux.[3] This makes sense, since if you have stomach juice contents in your throat, you have chemical sensors in your throat that make you wake up just enough to swallow. If there's additional air pressure in your throat, then it's more likely that with every swallow, you'll ingest some air. The more reflux you have, the more air you'll swallow. In this study, treating reflux helped the bloating symptoms.

One major reason for having throat reflux in the first place is persistent apneas. Tremendous vacuum forces are created in the chest and throat with each apnea or hypopnea. This forces your stomach contents up into your throat. As a result, you're more likely to swallow more often. This may be the reason why staying off your back has been found to lessen bloating while using CPAP. Since you're less likely to have apneas on your side, you won't swallow as often, and as a result, you'll have less air in your stomach.

Problem #10: Stuffy Nose

Forcing air through your nose can dry out your mucous membranes. Even with extra heated humidification, the additional flow of air can still dry your normal secretions.

Solution: Conservatively, using nasal saline sprays or irrigation can sometimes help. Many people with sleep apnea will have additional nasal congestion only when lying down. This is due to an involuntary system imbalance in your nose. Over-the-counter decongestant pills or sprays are not generally recommended. If standard medical treatment for allergies doesn't help, it's time to see an ear-nose-throat specialist to address your nasal congestion more definitively.

Some people will also have flimsy nostrils that cave in with nasal inhalation. You can try using one of the nasal dilator devices, such as Breathe Right® strips, which can be bought over-the-counter. There are also a number of options you can order online, such as Brez ™, Nozovent® and Sinus Cones®.

A much more detailed description of how you can un-stuff your stuffy nose can be found in Chapter 8.

Problem #11: Weight Gain While on CPAP

In general, sleeping better can promote weight loss, but a small proportion of CPAP users have been found to gain weight. A recent prospective randomized study involving 812 patients found that patients using CPAP were more likely to gain weight, as compared to patients on a sham CPAP over a six-month period.[4]

Solution: Many of my patients lose significant weight after starting CPAP, so this is a puzzling outcome. One possible explanation that was proposed in this study had to do with an imbalance in energy intake (EI) vs. energy expenditure (EE). OSA patients are thought to have higher energy expenditure during sleep. Therefore, by lowering EE by using CPAP at night, along with constant EI during the day, the resulting outcome may lead to weight gain. It's important to note that CPAP-adherent patients gained only about two pounds on average over six months.

If you feel that you've gained too much weight since starting CPAP, it's important to start a healthy exercise and diet program. You may need professional help, such as from a nutritionist or dietician. You'll have to decide if using CPAP is worth the benefits vs. the additional weight gain. This is a discussion you'll have to have with your sleep physician. If you gain a lot of weight, it's also important to make sure your CPAP pressure is adjusted properly, since pressure needs will rise with additional weight.

Problem #12: I Can't Fall Asleep

If you already have some degree of insomnia, then strapping a mask on to your face can definitely aggravate your insomnia problems.

Solution: In this situation, it's important to address all the issues that involve sleep hygiene. This includes not eating within three or four hours before bedtime, and not using any devices with an electronic screen before bedtime. A full list of steps for insomnia can be found by listening to my interview with Dr. Greg Jacobs, which you can find at doctorstevenpark. com/beatinsomnia. Worst-case scenario, your doctor may prescribe a short-term sleep aid to get you started. Going through the mask acclimation exercises may also help with this problem. I talk about this later in more detail in Chapter 9, *Your Seven Day CPAP Success Program.*

Problem #13: The Pressure is Too Strong

Having too much pressure is a common problem for many first-time CPAP users. It feels unnatural to sleep while air is being forced into your nose or mouth. In general, these forces are much lower than what's required for a hospital ventilator. For most people, with patience and a few helpful suggestions, success can be achieved.

Solution: The first tip is to use your machine's ramp feature. The pressure can be set to gradually increase to the final pressure over a predefined time period. Usually, this is over 20 minutes, but this setting can be changed. For example, if your pressure is 16 cm, your machine will start at 4 cm and gradually raise the pressure to 16 cm over 20 minutes. Ramping can be restarted if you haven't fallen asleep in those first 20 minutes. Over a period of a few weeks, you'll gradually get used to the pressure, and will be able to tolerate the therapy for longer periods of time.

Many of the newer machines have a pressure-relief function that lowers the applied pressure slightly as you start to breathe out. You can usually change the pressure level for this feature. C-Flex™, Bi-Flex® and EPR™ are some trademarked names for these features from various manufacturers.

In some cases, if ramping doesn't work, you can be switched to a bi-level PAP machine, which has a higher inhalation pressure set (that you were calibrated on), and a significantly lower exhalation pressure, so it's easier to breathe out.

Two Things That Go Flop In The Night

Since routinely performing endoscopy procedures during deep sleep, I've seen two interesting problems that can definitely prevent people from using CPAP. The first one is what I call expiratory palatal obstruction (EPO), when the soft palate flops back up into the nose during mid-nasal exhalation, causing a sudden blockage, with air leaking out through the mouth.

The second problem is when the epiglottis (the cartilaginous hood on top of your voice box) flops back quickly with each inhalation, causing sudden obstruction. This condition is more often seen in infants (called laryngomalacia), but can sometimes present in adults as well.

These obstructions may not last long enough to be picked up as an apnea or hypopnea during sleep studies. Sometimes these findings can be identified in the office, but most are seen in the operating room while under general anesthesia. In my experience, only surgery can help with these two conditions, allowing CPAP and even dental appliances to work much better. You can find example video clips of EPO and epiglottis collapse at doctorstevenpark.com/2things.

Problem #14: Skin Irritation

Skin irritation or breakdown is a common problem with CPAP masks. Temporary red marks or lines can be normal, but persistent red marks or peeled skin should be addressed immediately. This can usually be avoided by choosing a mask that fits properly, but even with the best-fitting masks, you can still suffer skin irritation.

Solution: Masks generally come in various sizes (small, medium and large). It's important to work with your DME technician to find a mask that not only fits well, but is also comfortable to use and has headgear that you like. Try adjusting the straps or repositioning the mask on your face. If you tried everything on your own and still have persistent marks or abrasions, it's time to call your DME to help you troubleshoot and possibly order a new mask.

The bridge of the nose is probably the most common area on the face for skin breakdown. People with a shallow nasal bridge will require masks that allow for this facial variation. Most manufacturers have fitting guides available, whether sold separately or within the packaging of the mask itself. If you continue to have skin problems, despite trying different nasal masks, then trying a nasal pillow type mask may be a good option as long as your machine's pressure is not too high. Some people switch back and forth between a nasal mask and a nasal pillow mask just to give their facial skin a chance to heal.

Another option that can be helpful is to use a mask liner. These devices form a barrier between your face and the mask, creating a better seal and lessening the possibility of skin irritation. There are numerous options that are available, made from different materials. A low-tech mask liner that some people have used is a Band-Aid® over the bridge of the nose. Product information can be found in the resources section at the end of this book.

In some cases, your straps may be too tight. Since most modern masks are designed to be applied to the face lightly, with pressure from the machine forming a tight seal, over-tightening can sometimes cause even more leaks. You may then mistakenly tighten the mask even more, causing more leaks, as well as causing more facial impressions and abrasions. Given that, in some cases, you may need to loosen your mask if you're having too much skin irritation.

If the mask or headgear straps are leaving marks on your face, I recommend looking at options available on CPAP supply websites such as Padacheek. com or Hope2Sleep.co.uk.

Problem #15: Water is Leaking from My Mask

When heated air passes through tubing in a colder room, water vapor can condensate. This is called rainout.

Solution: Here are your options to reduce or eliminate rainout:

1. Raise the room temperature.
2. Move your CPAP machine to a level below your head.
3. Insulate your hose.
4. Reduce the temperature setting on your heated humidifier.
5. Change to heated hosing.
6. Change to a CPAP unit that has built-in rainout reduction.

Summary

I often see patients who are very successful in the beginning, but stop using their machine because it simply stopped working as well as it used to. It turns out that by sleeping better, the patients naturally lost some weight.

Since their CPAP pressure was originally set for their original weight, the current pressure was too high, so CPAP wasn't working as well anymore. For whatever reason, no one thought to follow up six months later, and they ended up seeing me again years later. What was needed was a re-calibration of the CPAP pressure.

What I described above will probably cover 95% of all CPAP issues that arise. If there are questions that I haven't answered, your best resource is to ask the real CPAP experts: CPAP users themselves on sites like CPAPtalk. com, Hope2Sleep.co.uk or the American Sleep Apnea Association's Sleeptember forum.

Sinus Pain with CPAP

Ever since starting CPAP, I've had repeated sinus infections requiring multiple courses of antibiotics. I've never had sinus infections before. What can I do?

— John

Suffering from sinus pain, pressure and even infections is a common situation after starting CPAP. This can happen even if you keep the mask and tubing clean. One well-known phenomenon is what's called non-allergic, or chronic rhinitis, where the nervous system in your nose overreacts to weather changes, especially pressure changes. Adding unnatural levels of positive air pressure can definitely irritate the nose and sinus passageways, which can sometimes lead to inflammation. Swelling due to inflammation can lead to nasal or sinus congestion, and if prolonged, may lead to bacterial infections.

This is a difficult problem to treat, since this condition doesn't respond to allergy medications. However, some people do well with over-the-counter allergy medications and prescription allergy pills or sprays. Using lots of nasal saline sprays or irrigation can sometimes help. Experimenting with your CPAP's humidity settings may also help. Ultimately, if the problem becomes too severe, it's time to talk with your sleep doctor about trying something different. However, before you give up on CPAP, if your nose is stuffy, always consider optimizing your nasal breathing, whether through medications or even surgery.

Sometimes, pressure from CPAP can irritate the nasal and sinus passageways, causing a sinus migraine attack. This has to be treated like a migraine, in addition to the above recommendations.

More Helpful CPAP Tips

• • •

"Just do it."

—*Nike*

Jonathan, the college student, called me one day to tell me that he was going on a camping trip for three nights and wanted to know what his options were. Besides looking into getting a mandibular advancement device as a backup option, I gave him some advice about traveling with CPAP.

This chapter is made up of various additional topics and issues that people ask about. I've also included answers to the most common questions about CPAP that came in through my Ask Dr. Park teleseminars.

Cleaning Your CPAP

One of the biggest causes of anxiety in potential CPAP users is the regular cleaning that's required. Even cleaning your basic home humidifier every night can be a minor nuisance for some people. Most manufacturers recommend cleaning your mask every day—in the morning right after waking up is usually the best time. You don't need anything more than warm soapy water, using a mild detergent. Avoid antibacterial soaps, since some have alcohol, which can wear down the materials. Also, you should avoid soaps with fragrances or scents. Dove or Ivory liquid soaps are both good options. Let it air dry so that it's ready to be used at night.

The hose should be cleaned at least once every week. Running some soapy water through the hose in the shower or bath should suffice. You can also soak it in a basin for 15 to 30 minutes, then let it air dry. Running some white vinegar solution (one part vinegar, 10 parts water) through the hose on a monthly basis can also help disinfect the tubing. Make sure you flush it out with lots of water afterwards. The same recommendation applies to the water chamber for the heated humidifier. Since there may be variations in what each manufacturer recommends, it's important to read and follow your specific manual's directions.

All machines will also have a filter that will need to be changed. Your manual should tell you how often you need to do this.

All manufacturers will have their own cleaning and maintenance instructions, so it's important to read the instructions carefully.

Traveling with CPAP

Compared to even five years ago, traveling with CPAP is much easier these days. Transportation and Safety Administration (TSA) officers are now much more familiar with CPAP equipment, and there are clear guidelines on the TSA's website.[1] Let the TSA security officer know beforehand that you have a CPAP machine. They generally require that you take out the machine itself, but not the remaining accessories, such as the mask, headgear or tubing. You can provide a clear plastic bag to keep your machine clean during x-ray scanning. If necessary, you may have to remove the machine from the bag to check for traces of explosives.

There are different opinions on whether or not you should check your CPAP. Most people will carry it on the plane. If you do, it may count against your total number of carry-on items. Technically, it shouldn't be counted as a carry-on, since it's medical equipment. If you check it, however, make sure that's it's placed in a well-padded case.

If you plan on using CPAP onboard during a long flight, check with your carrier about CPAP use requirements, since every airline has different rules. Some carriers are more CPAP-friendly than others. Check to make sure that you have an outlet next to your seat, so you can use their AC power, or you may need to bring a battery pack. Having a letter from your doctor describing your condition is also not a bad idea, in case you run into an uninformed airline employee. Also, you should print out the TSA's ruling on CPAP and have it with you, just in case. Most frequent flyers who travel with CPAP will develop their own prophylactic routines, based on past experiences. Many CPAP models have available FAA compliance letters, which you'll be able to find on the manufacturer or retailer's websites.

Having an extension cord with a surge protector is also a good idea. This not only protects your device, but you'll also have more outlets for your computer, cell phone and other devices. Having a few extra fuses may also come in handy, just in case. Check and recheck to make sure that you're not forgetting anything before you leave your house.

If you travel outside the US, it's important to take a universal power adaptor with you. Make sure your machine can accommodate 110 and 220V. You should check the voltage levels of the country that you're traveling to before you leave, and also make sure that your CPAP's three-pronged plug will work with your adaptor. Be prepared to have a setup ready to suspend your hose above your head (from Chapter 4) if that's your normal routine.

Backup Battery Options

If you want a small, portable unit that will last through the night, there are a number of CPAP batteries that are sold online for about $300. It's important to check the power usage specification for your particular CPAP model, including the right type of adapters. The higher your machine's pressure, the more power it will use. Using heated humidification can use up to four times more power. There are many options available, ranging from very portable units to heavy-duty, longer-lasting units. If you're camping without electricity, solar power can also be used to recharge your CPAP battery. More information and prices can easily be found on product information pages online.

There are a lot of creative CPAP users that have demonstrated less expensive options. One simple solution is to use a portable multipurpose battery from Sears for around $150. This battery can even be recharged using your car's cigarette lighter while you're driving. If you're handy with electronics, you can build a CPAP battery system using a car battery. Specific instructions can be found if you search for 'CPAP camping' on YouTube. This option will give you a few nights of CPAP use at best without recharging. If you choose to try this, consult with an electrician and proceed at your own risk.

CPAP Machine Location

Should you place it on your nightstand or on the floor? There's no right answer to this question, with advantages and disadvantages to both locations. Placing it on the floor can lessen the noise issue, but it will get a bit dustier, especially around the air intake vents. You'll also have fewer rainout episodes with the machine on the floor. However, having an electronic device on the floor is generally not advisable, particularly if you have to vacuum the carpet or rug around your device. In this situation, placing it on top of a short stand is probably a better idea.

Placing it on your nightstand will give you more slack in your tubing. However, there are reports of machines being pulled off nightstands due to excessive tube tension while the user turns in bed. Placing a rubbery anti-slip mat underneath your machine will not only keep it more securely fastened, but can also dampen any noise.

Some people place their machines inside their nightstand drawers with holes cut out in the back for the tubing and electrical lines. You can even purchase CPAP nightstands. This will also dampen any noise. During the day, you can't see the CPAP machine at all. Ultimately, you'll have to experiment to find the best location for you.

Going to the Bathroom, Made Easier

It's generally recommended to keep your mask on when you have to go to the bathroom in the middle of the night. This way, you don't have to adjust your mask in the dark before going back to sleep. You may struggle to remove the tubing from the mask, and coming back to bed can be another struggle, particularly trying to reattach the tube to your mask in the dark while you're half asleep. If this happens to you, there's a simple adaptor that makes the coupling/uncoupling process much easier. It's so quick and easy that you can literally do it with one hand. Most CPAP supply stores or your DME company should carry it in stock. If you prefer to take off your mask, then this is a moot point.

Cover the Lights

Most modern electronic devices have extra bright lights on the control panels. In some cases, they can be even brighter than night-lights. It's a good idea to cover these lights on your CPAP machine, as well as on the other devices in your bedroom. Having light in your room lowers melatonin production and can prevent sleep onset. You can place something in front of your machine, or use black electrical tape to cover the lights.

Sabbath Considerations

CPAP users who observe the Sabbath have a number of different options. You can talk to your rabbi and get it sanctioned, since it's a potentially a life-threatening health condition. You can turn it on before Sabbath begins and place the mask on when you go to bed. You can then turn it off once Sabbath ends. However, this may skew your adherence data. A separate timer has also been recommended, but most CPAP machines won't start blowing automatically when the power is turned on. The best course of action is to talk with your sleep physician, rabbi, or DME professional to come up with a reasonable plan.

Undergoing Surgery

If you're undergoing surgery or have to be admitted to the hospital for an overnight stay, take your CPAP machine with you. For mild cases of sleep apnea, you can go a day or two without CPAP, but if you have moderate or severe sleep apnea, it's important to use CPAP during your stay. There are two reasons for this. First, you'll sleep much better. Second, using CPAP may lessen the chances of complications during your hospital stay, especially if you have to undergo anesthesia for an endoscopy or need to stay overnight. This is especially important if you are forced to sleep on your back and if you require pain medications (which can potentially lower your drive to breathe).

If you don't take your machine with you, it's likely that the hospital will place you on a regular respirator set to straight CPAP or bi-level settings. They also won't have your particular mask and headgear. Furthermore, it's unlikely to have built-in adjustable levels of humidification. In my experience, few hospitals are familiar with consumer CPAP devices that are used outside of a hospital setting, so you'll have to take some responsibility for your own care.

It's important to talk with your surgeon or physician about these issues if you're a regular CPAP user. If you're undergoing nasal or facial surgery, it may prevent CPAP use while you're recovering for a period of time.

What is the Smallest and Lightest CPAP Machine?

CPAP models are constantly changing, but as of writing this book, the smallest CPAP machine I know of is the Z1 from *Human Design Medical*. It weighs only 10 ounces and measures about 6.5 x 3.3 x 2 inches. It's also very quiet at only 26 decibels. A portable battery pack is available, and it can be used as a travel machine or as a regular machine. Note that it doesn't include a humidifier.

As of this book's writing, there's news of an extremely small micro-CPAP device called Airng™. It seems like it's currently in early phases of development and will require FDA approval.

How Often Do You Need to Re-check the Pressure or Calibrate Your Machine?

If your machine is not working like it used to, or if you've gained or lost a significant amount of weight, you may want to re-calibrate your pressure. It's also a good idea to think about re-calibrating every 6-12 months, even if you're doing well. Most sleep doctors will want you to come back and undergo another in-lab CPAP titration. Some physicians will manually adjust your pressure up or down by a few notches, depending on how you're feeling, without doing another sleep study. With newer data-reporting machines, it's easy to see whether or not you need to change your pressure. If you think that your machine is defective or unable to maintain a prescribed pressure, check with your sleep lab or DME company. They have pressure-reading devices that can check your machine for you.

Many people stop using CPAP after a few months or years because they find that it doesn't work as well as it did in the past. This is a big mistake. If this happens, it's time to consider readjusting the pressure.

Can I Change the Pressure Myself?

The official answer given by the sleep medical community is a firm "No." The first argument is that it's similar to changing the dosage or frequency of a prescribed medication without your doctor's orders. Secondly, it could also cause central apneas if the pressure is too high.

However, there are certain situations where you may decide to take control of your pressure setting. I've known many patients that have become experts in their own care, sometimes being even more proficient than the sleep doctor. By reading the data that's reported and adjusting the pressures as needed, this is doable, but only if you have the technical skills and the motivation to do this. For example, one patient I know adjusts his pressure a bit higher whenever his nose is stuffy due to allergies or a cold. Once the congestion is better, he lowers the pressure back to his normal baseline.

The fact that you can make changes, look at the data, and simultaneously correlate the effect with how you feel on a day-to-day basis is a major advantage. Getting the doctor to place the order to the DME, who will then arrange to change your machine pressure, can take days to weeks. For those of you who are given APAP machines, this is not as much of an issue, since your pressure is being adjusted automatically.

In all cases, this process must be monitored on a regular basis with a sleep physician. I predict that with online data reporting, along with some of the newer smartphone or computer applications that can provide real-time data, we can all work together with more efficient and effective results.

Can I Test Out Masks for CPAP Machines?

Since CPAP masks must touch your face, they cannot be reused by other people. Hopefully, following a proper fitting by your sleep care team, you won't need more than one mask. However, if you do need to try a different mask, let your DME company know within 30 days. Otherwise, you'll have to pay for a new one, or wait 90 days for a replacement.

Do I Have to Use CPAP When Taking a Nap?

In general, the answer is yes, but there are a few exceptions. If you take a very short nap, it's unlikely that you'll ever enter REM sleep, which is when all your muscles relax. Also, if you only have mild sleep apnea, then it's probably not worth using CPAP every time you take a nap. However, if you take naps that are longer than 30 to 45 minutes, using CPAP is recommended.

Can I Use CPAP When My Nose is Stuffy Due to a Cold or Allergies?

Yes, you can, but it just won't work as well. Some simple steps you can take include irrigating with nasal saline, or taking an over-the-counter decongestant pill or spray. It's important not to use decongestant sprays, like Afrin® or any nasal decongestant containing the ingredient oxymetazoline, for more than two or three days. If you have allergies, you can take over-the-counter medications or antihistamines, or see your doctor for prescription allergy medications if you need something stronger.

Will I Have to Use Humidification All Year Round?

At least some amount of humidification is generally recommended, but in certain humid environments, humidification may not be necessary. It all depends on your individual needs and your sleep environment. Some people do better without humidification. The only way to tell is to experiment and figure out what works best.

Can I Use My CPAP at High Altitudes?

Most modern CPAP machines, especially ones with data capability, will compensate automatically, but only up to about 8,000 feet. On some older CPAP models, you also may have to change the settings manually, depending on your elevation level. If you have to go much higher than that, talk to your sleep physician about making the necessary pressure adjustments, or perhaps even adding oxygen to your therapy. In theory, an APAP may be a better option if you have to frequently travel to high elevations.

Can I Sleep on My Side Using CPAP?

It may be more challenging, but it is possible to sleep on your side. There are a number of different pillows that can help you sleep comfortably on your side. Certain CPAP masks are also more amenable to side sleeping. This also depends on the shape, size, and configuration of your tubing. With the right equipment, some experimentation and persistence, you should be able to use CPAP on your side.

Can I Use CPAP if I Have a Beard?

Any contact of the mask interface with facial hair may promote air leaks or require a tighter fit.

However, you can absolutely use CPAP. Your first choice should be to use a nasal pillow type of interface, but if your pressure is on the high side, you may need to switch to a regular nasal or full-face mask. Any contact of your mask with facial hair may promote leakage or require a tighter fit (which can make things worse).

There are a number of masks that are more amenable to men with beards. Talk with your DME representative or online sources for the best current models. Worst-case scenario, you may need to shave off your mustache or beard.

Whom Do You Call for Help?

One common question that I get is who a successful CPAP user should call when they need replacement parts. In most cases, you'll have a sleep physician and a durable medical equipment (DME) company. Sometimes, you may also have an otolaryngologist (ENT) or dentist involved. In most cases, the sleep physician works inside the sleep lab where you underwent your sleep study, but not always. In some cases, it's the otolaryngologist that orders the sleep study and orders your CPAP. It can get very confusing.

If your sleep physician handled everything, then call the sleep physician for any issues that you may have, including technical issues, such as needing a replacement mask or PAP supplies. He or she will need to write an order to the DME. Calling your DME will delay things, since the DME will have to contact the ordering physician.

If you have multiple doctors taking care of you, keep track of who ordered your CPAP machine. However, for problem solving or technical issues with your CPAP machine, calling your DME is the first step. If you haven't already done this, place a sticker with your CPAP ordering physician and your DME company phone number on the back of your CPAP machine. I can't tell you how many times people forget who to call, since they may not need to make a call for a year or two.

How Long Do CPAP Machines Last?

With proper care, most machines should last at least five years. In fact, some people have used their machines for over ten years. Most machines are covered under a manufacturer's warranty for about three years. Insurance companies will usually allow machine replacement or upgrades every three to five years. If it's broken, insurance will usually cover the replacement or repair costs. If you purchase it outright, then you're out of luck after the warranty period is over.

Summary

As a surgeon, I love to solve problems. Whether it's working on household problems, my car, patient health issues, or even handling the occasional disagreements that come up with my wife, my first initial reaction to any problem is, "How can I fix it?"

This knee-jerk reaction is also my downfall. I'm very good at fixing immediate problems that arise, but similar issues seem to keep coming back. For example, for someone with a mouth leak, one common recommendation is to switch to a full-face mask. This often works, but the basic problem often still remains: a stuffy nose. By treating your stuffy nose with medicines or surgery, not only will you breathe better, the CPAP will work better and your pressures may even be lowered. I'm sure that in various relationship issues, the same concept also applies. What's the underlying reason for the disagreement or problem? Is there something that's blocked or bottled up that needs to be addressed before applying a quick fix that won't last?

Jonathan, as an electrical engineer, was ecstatic that solar-powered battery systems for CPAP were available. Since he was going camping on a beach, the idea seemed perfect. He began designing his own homemade system. With the right knowledge-based resources and with his resourcefulness, he was determined not to let a camping trip prevent him from getting a great night's sleep. He also agreed to look into getting an oral appliance made as another backup option.

The past few chapters have likely covered 95% of the issues that arise when using CPAP. I'm amazed how resourceful some people can be when they go to great lengths to optimize their CPAP experience. One patient modified his mask using duct tape to create a better seal. I also mentioned Bruce Stein's book (*Sleep Apnea and CPAP - A User's Manual by a User*), where he explains how to suspend your hose above your head to prevent mask leaks.

The next chapter will cover one of the most important things you should do before ever trying CPAP: how to un-stuff your stuffy nose.

CHAPTER 8

Un-stuff Your Stuffy Nose

• • •

"To know even one life has breathed easier because
you have lived. This is to have succeeded."

—RALPH WALDO EMERSON

PETER IS A 50-YEAR-OLD FIREMAN who was referred to me by his sleep physician, since he could not stand using CPAP at night. He kept ripping off the mask within two to three hours of falling asleep. His insurance company was asking him to return his CPAP machine due to non-compliance issues. During the initial consultation, I noted that his nasal septum was so crooked that it was actually touching the left sidewall of his nose. He mentioned that he had been given allergy pills and sprays by his allergist years ago for his stuffy nose, but that they didn't help. Peter was expecting me to offer surgical options for his sleep apnea, since I'm a surgeon.

For the vast majority of you that have similar issues, my first recommendation is usually not throat surgery, but rather making sure that you're able to breathe properly through your nose. I mentioned in prior chapters that having open nasal passageways can significantly improve your chances of being able to use and benefit from CPAP. The one study I cite found that nasal surgery increased CPAP use from 30 minutes to over five hours.

Having a stuffy nose will cause you to open your mouth, which can aggravate mouth leaks, lowering the pressure that's delivered to your throat, and aggravating more apneas. Even if you have a full-face mask (that covers your nose and mouth), opening your mouth can still lead to leaks. Full-face masks typically require higher pressures, which makes CPAP less comfortable, in general. The good news is that nasal surgery has also been found to lower CPAP pressures for many people.

Your nose and sinuses also produce a gas called nitric oxide. This gas is produced in small amounts, but when inhaled into the lungs, it significantly enhances your lung's capacity to absorb oxygen (about 10 to 25%). Nitric oxide is also lethal to bacteria and viruses, which is why it's generally important to inhale through your nose.

In this chapter, I start with the basics, describing conservative measures to medical therapy and, if needed, which nasal surgery might work for you. Even if medications and non-surgical options work, some people would rather not have to take medication for the rest of their lives.

Again, it's also important to mention that nasal surgery has not been found to be helpful in treating obstructive sleep apnea. The main reason for offering nasal surgery is to help patients breathe much better nasally. As a potential side benefit, you may be able to use CPAP much more effectively. Good nasal breathing is very important for many reasons, which is why I want to cover this topic a bit more extensively. For more information, you can download a copy of my free e-book Un-stuff Your Stuffy Nose at doctorstevenpark.com

Nasal Anatomy Lesson

Before I discuss the various ways to breathe better, a short anatomy lesson is in order. The nasal septum is a thin sheet of cartilage and bone that splits your nasal cavity right down the middle. No one has a perfectly straight

78

septum; everyone's septum is slightly curved. Sometimes, nasal trauma can shift or move the septum away from its midline position. The nasal turbinates are wing-like structures that line the sidewalls of your nose. The sidewall is covered with a mucous membrane layer, which normally helps to smooth, warm and humidify air. The turbinates and sinuses also produce about two pints of mucous every day. Turbinates normally swell and shrink, alternating from side to side every few hours. This is called the nasal cycle.

The front sidewalls make up your nostrils, which are soft pieces of cartilage that are covered on the inside with mucous membranes and the outside with skin. The back of your nose is one big cavity (called the nasopharynx), and the passageway turns down 90 degrees into the back of your throat. The nasopharynx is also where your ears connect via the Eustachian tubes.

If any part of the anatomy that I described becomes blocked, either partially or completely, you'll feel stuffy in your nose. Usually, it's not one thing, but rather a combination of different reasons. For example, if you have a mildly deviated septum, allergies will swell up your nasal turbinates, and narrow your nasal passageways. This may not be enough to clog up your nose, but if you have flimsy nostrils or had a rhinoplasty in the past that weakened the nostrils, then breathing in with a stuffy nose may trigger your nostrils to collapse.

Here are seven basic conservative, nonsurgical steps you can take to enjoy better nasal breathing:

#1: Do you have flimsy nostrils?

Starting from the tip of your nose, the first thing you must do is find out whether you have flimsy nostrils. If you have a very narrow nose, or if your nostril openings are very narrow and slit-like, then you may be likely to have flimsy nostrils. Try this experiment: Take both index fingers and press them just besides your nostrils on your cheek. While firmly pressing on your cheeks, lift the cheek skin upwards and sideways, toward the outer corners of your eyes. Take a deep breath in. Can you breathe much better through your nose? Let go and try it again. If this maneuver does improve your breathing, then you may benefit from using nasal dilator strips at night (one common brand is called Breathe Right®). Sometimes, the adhesive on these strips is not strong enough, or they end up irritating the skin. Another way of treating this condition is to use various internal dilator devices that you can find over the counter or online (e.g., Nozovent®, Sinus Cones®).

#2: NASAL SALINE SPRAYS OR IRRIGATION

Second, try using nasal saline sprays. You can use the simple spray bottles that put out a fine mist, more sophisticated methods like aerosol cans, or even a Water-Pik machine (there's a nasal adaptor that you can buy for this). Another popular variation is something called a Neti Pot, which uses a teapot-like container to pour salt water into your nose and sinuses and uses gravity to clear you up.

You can either use prepared saline packages found in most pharmacies or mix your own recipe (one cup of boiled lukewarm water and 1/2 teaspoon of sea salt or Kosher salt with a pinch of baking soda). Do not use table salt, since it can include additives. You can use an infant nasal bulb syringe, a turkey baster syringe, or a large medical syringe (without the needle). It's important to wash whatever you use to irrigate your nose with soap and hot water in order to avoid contamination.

Whatever method you use, you'll have to do it frequently for maximum results. Besides cleaning out mucous, pollutants and allergens, saline also acts as a mild decongestant.

#3: Avoid eating within three to four hours of sleep

Don't eat anything within three hours of going to bed. If you still have food or juices lingering in your stomach when you go to bed, it can passively leak up into your throat, not only preventing a good night's sleep, but also leaking up into your nose, causing swelling and inflammation. In addition, many people will also stop breathing once in a while, which creates a vacuum effect in the throat that actively suctions up your stomach juices into your throat and nose.

#4: Avoid alcohol near bedtime

Try to avoid drinking alcohol close to bedtime. Not only does alcohol irritate the stomach, but it also relaxes your throat muscles as you sleep, which aggravates the process described in the previous paragraph.

#5: Control your allergies

If you have any known allergies, especially if it's an allergy to something in your bedroom, try to either remove it or lessen your exposure. For example, if you have carpeting or an area rug, it can harbor dust or animal dander. Frequently washing your bed sheets in very hot water also helps. Investing in a quality HEPA filter should help even more. If you have any pets, consider keeping them out of your bedroom. If conservative measures to control allergies don't work, consider over-the-counter allergy medications.

There are various over-the-counter allergy medications available. The newer, non-sedating antihistamines block the effects of histamine, which is what causes watery, itchy, runny eyes and noses. The most common brands are Claritin®, Allegra® and Zyrtec®. They all work differently for different people, so the only thing you can do is try each one and see which you prefer. Although they are non-sedating in theory, there are reported cases of drowsiness with all three. Claritin® and Allegra® are the least potentially sedating, but Zyrtec® is slightly more likely to make you drowsy. Benadryl® is an older antihistamine that's very effective for allergies, except many more people may get drowsy.

If your nose is stuffy, another option you can try is a nasal decongestant spray like Afrin® (main ingredient is oxymetazoline). However, you can only use this for two-three days, as this can be addictive. Pills for nasal congestion include the ingredients pseudoephedrine or phenylephrine, which can cause you to be jittery or overly stimulated. People with high blood pressure or prostate problems may want to avoid using these medications. Routine nasal saline irrigation can also help with your nasal allergies.

There are a number of prescription medications, including topical nasal steroids or antihistamine sprays. Leukotriene phosphate blockers, such as Singulair®, are another option. This is also used for asthma symptoms. Oral steroids like prednisone can also be useful in emergency situations. As a last resort, an allergy evaluation with immunotherapy (allergy shots) should be a consideration.

Regardless of how you treat your allergies, it's important to follow all these recommendations for better breathing while sleeping. Having a stuffy nose for any reason can trigger breathing pauses downstream, ultimately giving you a poor night's sleep.

#6: Exercise your nose

Get regular exercise, especially outdoors. Not only are you exercising your heart and your muscles, but you're also exercising the nervous system in your nose. Vigorous physical activity activates your sympathetic nervous system, which constricts the blood vessels that supply your nasal turbinates.

#7: LOWER STRESS

Lastly, slow down and relax. Modern society has removed all the natural built-in breaks throughout the day. Along with the information overload and constant stimulation, going nonstop all day only adds to the increased stress levels that everyone experiences. Between major activities, take a minute or so to stop what you're doing and stretch, get up, move around, and do some deep-breathing exercises. Stress can cause the muscles to tense up, causing you to take shallower breaths, which results in physiologic changes that can ultimately aggravate nasal congestion.

If you have tried all the above-mentioned conservative and medical options for your stuffy nose, and nothing helps, then surgery may be a good option for you. This section will describe surgical options for the three most common conditions that cause nasal congestion that I see in my practice: deviated nasal septum, enlarged turbinates, and flimsy nostrils. There are many other reasons for nasal congestion, including chronic sinusitis and adenoid enlargement, but those are beyond the scope of this book. A thorough evaluation by your otolaryngologist (ENT surgeon) is important to determine what's causing your nasal breathing problems.

MYTHS AND FACTS ABOUT SEPTOPLASTY

A septoplasty operation is one of the procedures most misunderstood by lay people – and even many physicians. Some people only equate septoplasty with having a cosmetic rhinoplasty, which is not true. However, there are people who *do* use having a deviated septum as an excuse to undergo a rhinoplasty. What follows is a brief description of septal anatomy, when a septoplasty is required, a brief review of the surgical technique, and what to expect after the surgery.

First of all, the nasal septum is the midline cartilaginous structure that divides the two halves of your nasal cavity. The parts in the back of the septum are made of bone. Whenever the septum is crooked to a significant degree, your nose can become stuffy easily, and a septoplasty can be offered if conservative options don't work.

However, having a crooked septum doesn't mean that you'll have a stuffy nose or that you'll need a septoplasty. No one has a perfectly straight septum. There are a number of other parts of your nasal anatomy that contribute to your ability to breathe, which I will cover in this chapter.

It's often taught that trauma is the most common reason for a deviated nasal septum. Pressure from leaving the birth canal or being punched in the nose are common explanations. However, people who are born via C-section can still have a severely deviated nasal septum.

The simplest explanation is that modern human jaws are shrinking due to what we eat and how we eat. Eating soft foods, bottle-feeding, thumb-sucking, pacifier use, prematurity and nasal congestion are all risk factors for crooked teeth (malocclusion). Having crooked teeth means that your jaws are not big enough to hold all your teeth. In more severe cases, the roof of your mouth (hard palate) doesn't drop normally during development. This leads to the narrowing of your dental arches, resulting in smaller oral cavity volumes and crowding of the soft tissues inside your mouth. This is a proposed explanation for obstructive sleep apnea.

Inside your nose, if the floor of your nose doesn't drop as your nasal septum grows, it will buckle to one side instead, leading to a deviated nasal septum. Additionally, the sidewalls of your nose will be closer to the midline, since they follow your narrower upper molars. The angle between your septum and fleshy nostrils is also more narrow, which pre-disposes them to caving in whenever you inhale.

What's Involved with Septal Surgery?

There are many ways to perform a septoplasty, but the most important point is that it should be done well, no matter which approach is used. The septum is covered on both sides by a mucous membrane, and after an incision is made inside the nose on the mucous membrane, this layer is peeled away from the septal cartilage. The other side of the nose is also entered, which creates two tunnels on either side of the septal cartilage. Next, the crooked part of the septal cartilage is removed. Some surgeons either soften the cartilage or flatten it out and put it back, while others leave it out completely. In some cases, a small portion of the bony spur that juts out at the base of the septal cartilage is also removed.

The last part of the operation is where different surgeons use different techniques. Traditionally, thin plastic sheets with or without soft sponge-like packs are placed against the septum on both sides to keep the mucous membrane together for proper healing. If a large clot of blood forms between the two mucous membrane layers, the remaining cartilage may lose its blood supply and literally melt away. This can lead to what's called a saddle-nose deformity, where you see a mild depression in the external, middle part of your nose. This is why splints or packs are often used.

The surgical steps that I describe are my personal preferences. Other surgeons may use different techniques. Because the entire procedure is done inside the nose, there is no swelling, bruising or changes to the outside of the nose or face, unless a rhinoplasty is done at the same time.

What to Expect After Septum Surgery

If packs are used, they are removed anywhere from one to five days after the surgery. Many patients report that this is one of the most uncomfortable parts of undergoing this procedure. Some surgeons, like myself, don't use any packs or splints. Instead, I use the following method: compressing the two mucous membrane layers by sewing the two layers together using a dissolvable suture, like a quilting stitch. A septal stapler can also be used. This way, nothing needs to be removed, and you can breathe much better right after the surgery. With this procedure, it's expected that your nose will become clogged up after a day or two with an accumulation of blood, mucous and debris. This is usually cleaned out in the office on your first post-operative visit.

This operation is usually performed as an outpatient procedure, so you'll go home a few hours after the surgery. It's usually performed under general anesthesia, but can also be done with local anesthesia and sedation for certain situations. Most people can go back to work after two or three days. Heavy straining or lifting should be avoided for about one week.

In my practice, I see patients about three to five days after the surgery, and make sure the nose is cleaned of all the accumulated mucous and blood. Some people need a second cleaning one to two weeks later. Frequent nasal saline irrigation is strongly recommended to prevent the build-up of crusting. Gentle nose blowing is allowed, especially after nasal saline irrigation.

Typically, it may take a few weeks to months to feel the full benefits of this operation. During the first few weeks, crusts will build up and fall out as the wounds heal. This is also when the swelling from the surgery goes away. Afterwards, scarring and tightening of the soft tissues can take weeks to months. You may have your ups and downs in the first few weeks, but you should see consistent improvement by three to four weeks.

Most people can get by with over-the-counter pain medications such as Tylenol® or Advil®, but a prescription narcotic medication is prescribed just in case. You'll probably be more bothered by the sore throat caused by having a breathing tube placed.

What Are the Risks?

Complications are rare, but with any surgical procedure, there is a small chance of infection or bleeding. There is also a small risk any time someone undergoes general anesthesia, which includes allergic or medication reactions, as well as airway problems. In terms of overall risk, it's riskier when you cross the street in New York City. Other very rare potential complications include the loss of your sense of smell, a hole in your septum, or saddle-nose deformity.

A septoplasty, if done properly, is one of the most gratifying procedures for both patients and surgeons. Success rates are very high, but in a small percentage of patients, nasal congestion still persists, or it comes back after a few weeks to months. In this situation, there are three main possible reasons: the septum was not addressed aggressively enough, there is persistent turbinate swelling due to inflammation, or you have flimsy nostrils. Fortunately, there are treatment options for all these conditions.

The Turbinates: What You Should Know

Most people know about the septum and sinuses when it comes to breathing, but far fewer people know about the nasal turbinates. Turbinates are like wings along the sidewalls of your nasal cavity, opposite your midline nasal septum. There are three paired structures: the inferior, middle and superior turbinates. Your sinus passageways drain from underneath the middle turbinates. Swollen turbinates are probably responsible for most cases of nasal congestion.

The turbinates are bony on the inside and surrounded by a mucous membrane covering, with very rich vascular tissue in between. The vascular tissue can engorge significantly, similar to what occurs with the penis. Any degree of inflammation, irritation or infection can aggravate turbinate swelling, and allergies are a very common cause. Even weather changes such as temperature, pressure or humidity fluctuations can aggravate turbinate swelling.

Sometimes it's difficult to tell whether a swollen structure is a turbinate or a polyp. A polyp is a protuberance of mucous membrane that grows beyond the normal tissue boundaries. Most nasal polyps originate from beneath the middle turbinates where the sinuses drain, but polyps can also occur anywhere in the nose, including on the turbinates.

Gravity also affects the size of your nasal turbinates. When you lie down, blood pools in the vessels, leading to their slight engorgement. However, your involuntary nervous system detects this relative change and automatically constricts your blood vessels to improve breathing. The same process occurs when you exercise—due to activation of the sympathetic nervous system, the turbinates shrink, opening up your breathing passageways.

Sometimes, the balance between the two halves of the involuntary nervous system (the sympathetic and parasympathetic parts) is out of alignment, meaning that this automatic mechanism doesn't work properly. Therefore, when you lie down or exercise, the vessels don't constrict fully. Other times, the turbinates become extra sensitive to allergies, weather changes, chemicals, scents or odors. Once it's irritated, an inflammatory reaction occurs that leads to engorgement and the production of mucous. This is called vasomotor or non-allergic rhinitis. Throat acid reflux has also been shown to be associated with this condition.

Ultimately, how well you breathe through your nose is determined by a combination of the size of your turbinates, your septal geometry, and how flimsy your nostrils are (see earlier sections on the septum and flimsy nostrils.) Your nose is not just a passive tube that acts a channel for air to pass into the lungs—it's a very dynamic structure, able to change minute by minute.

What You Must Know About Turbinate Surgery

If you've tried all the conservative options for treating your allergies or nasal congestion, and surgery is the only option left, there are a few very important facts you should know before undergoing any type of turbinate surgery. Decades ago, surgeons used to completely remove the inferior nasal turbinates. Initially, patients would breathe much better, but years later, they would complain of

> **Turbinate Trivia**
>
> One important feature of the turbinates that few people know about is what's called the nasal cycle. The turbinates alternate in size from side to side every few hours. One side shrinks and the other side swells. Normally, you won't notice this, unless both your turbinates are somewhat congested. If you have a deviated septum, you'll be more aware of this constant flux.

either a dry nose, a constantly runny nose, or even a return of nasal congestion. Paradoxically, when you look into these patient's noses, the nasal cavity would be wide open. This phenomenon is called the empty nose syndrome (ENS). Fortunately, this complete removal is rarely performed these days.

We now know that turbinates are a vital part of your nasal anatomy and function, and that you need a certain amount of nasal resistance to sense proper breathing. Surgeons now try to preserve as much of the turbinates as possible, especially the mucous membranes.

There are a variety of options for shrinking nasal turbinates, from conservative approaches to more aggressive ones. The simplest procedure that can be performed in the office is a cautery procedure. This is where a needle or probe is placed underneath the mucous membranes and the blood vessels are either cauterized or vaporized using electrical or radio-frequency energy. Over time, the scar tissue that's created shrinks and tightens the turbinate soft tissues. You'll see various names for approaches and techniques, such as radio frequency or Somnoplasty®.

One recent variation called Coblation® uses radio-frequency energy to vaporize tissues at relatively low temperatures. All these procedures have the advantage that they can be performed in the office, and no cutting or excising of the mucous membrane is involved.

The remaining procedures are usually performed in the operating room, under local or general anesthesia. There are many ways that surgeons modify, shrink, de-bulk, or excise parts of the turbinate. The previously mentioned in-office procedures can be performed, along with any other procedures, such as a septoplasty or sinus surgery. The simplest way is to physically cut the front-lower portion of the turbinate off using scissors or electrocautery. The deep bony parts are sometimes removed as well. These days, lasers are rarely used.

Another popular method is called a sub-mucous resection (meaning that any deep bone, cartilage or tissue is removed, leaving the overlying mucous membrane behind). For the turbinates, an incision is made lengthwise along the lower portion of the inferior turbinate, the bone is exposed and a portion is removed. The mucous membrane layers are replaced and pressed down onto the raw bony bed with soft nasal packing. A more updated way of doing this without making an incision is to use what's called a suction microdebrider, a device that has been used for years in sinus surgery. The tip of a long thin rod with an open end has a rotating blade that moves back and forth, while applying a vacuum to suction out whatever tissue is removed (either soft tissue or bone).

What to Expect After Turbinate Surgery

Many surgeons still use nasal packing, especially during more aggressive procedures, to keep the mucous membrane layer pressed against the raw surfaces. Since turbinate procedures are usually performed alongside septal procedures, nasal packing with or without splints is more common than not. Depending on each surgeon's preference, packing may or may not be used for minimally invasive procedures.

Turbinate procedures by themselves are not considered painful. Most patients don't take any pain medications unless other procedures are performed simultaneously.

It may take anywhere from days to weeks before your breathing improves significantly, since there will be an accumulation of blood and mucous immediately after the procedure. Many surgeons clean out this debris a few days to a week after the procedure during the follow-up appointment. Nasal saline can be applied every few hours for a few days after the surgery to loosen the secretions. Blowing your nose is typically discouraged, but for most of my patients I encourage gentle nose-blowing after applying nasal saline.

Turbinate surgery is a very useful procedure that can be done alone or in combination with other procedures. Bleeding and infection, although rare, can occur, just like with any other surgical procedure. There can also be anesthesia risks. In the rare case that the procedure fails, the reasons for failure include it being too conservative of a procedure, persistent nasal septal deviation, or nasal valve collapse.

Do You Have Flimsy Nostrils?

The other structure that is often overlooked is your nostrils. For most people, inhaling causes a mild vacuum effect that causes a mild collapse and constriction of the nostrils. However, in some people with either flimsy or weakened nostrils (from prior rhinoplasty), they fall in very easily, with even the slightest bit of inhalation. Unfortunately, many people undergo a number of different medical treatments using allergy sprays or even surgery before this condition of flimsy nostrils is even considered. If you are one of these people, as mentioned earlier in this chapter, you may benefit from nasal dilator strips (Breathe Right® is one brand). Sometimes, these strips are not strong enough or they can irritate the skin. Another option is to use internal nasal dilators, which tend to work much better. Some of the more common brands are Sinus Cones® and Nozovent®.

There are three simple ways to tell if you have flimsy nostrils:

1. Look in the mirror and take a deep breath through your nose. Do the sidewalls of your nostrils cave in as you breathe in?
2. Place your index finger just beside your nostrils on both sides. While pushing gently on each side, pull the cheek skin up and away from the nose, toward the outer corners of your eyes. Breathe in and see how you feel.
3. Using the back end of two Q-Tips®, place the thin end inside your nostril and lift up and sideways. Take a deep breath in. Is your breathing noticeably improved?

One very important point to make here is that how stuffy your nose is on the inside can also determine how much your nostrils will collapse. Think of it as sucking through a flimsy straw. If you pinch the middle slowly, the distant end of the straw will cave in since there's increased airflow. The same thing happens with your nostrils. In many cases, properly addressing nasal allergies or a deviated septum and enlarged turbinates will prevent your nostrils from caving in.

If you use over-the-counter decongestants like Afrin® or Sudafed® and you can breathe much better, then you should address the inside of your nose first. However, if you still have nasal congestion and it's obvious that your nostrils are caving in, then you may need to address this area as well.

NOSTRIL SURGERY

The most common way of managing flimsy nostrils surgically is through a functional nasal reconstruction procedure, using rhinoplasty techniques. This often has to be done through what's called an open rhinoplasty approach, where a small incision is made at the bottom of your nose and the cut is continued inside the nostrils on both sides. The skin is peeled off the lower half of the nose to expose the flimsy cartilage. A cartilage graft taken from your septum or ear is placed on top of the exposed sidewall cartilage and the skin is placed back down and closed. There can be a little widening of your nose due to added support structures.

There are also a number of ways to tighten your nostrils from the inside only. One technique that I like is to make a slight cut on the inner sidewalls of your nostrils, between two named pieces of cartilage (the upper and lower lateral cartilage). On the outside, you can see the crease or indentation where these two cartilage structures meet. You may see how it caves in during nasal inhalation. The two cartilages are separated off the skin through the cut from inside the nose, overlapped a few millimeters, and then tied down using a dissolvable stitch. It's like a mild nose-lift from the inside. As it heals over a few weeks or months, the nostrils stiffen. You will have some swelling for a few weeks. In theory, you can have a very slight widening of your nostrils, but in most cases you won't see anything noticeable after a few months.

Peter, the fireman mentioned earlier in this chapter, eventually elected to undergo septoplasty, turbinoplasty and nasal valve repair procedures for his nasal congestion. He understood that nasal surgery alone was not likely to get rid of his sleep apnea. Two months later, not only was he breathing much better through his nose, but he was also able to use CPAP much more effectively. His CPAP pressure needed to be lowered and he didn't have as many air leaks through his mouth. His sleep quality improved so much that he felt like he was 20 years old again.

CPAP Success and Beyond

• • •

"Success is the sum of small efforts, repeated day in and day out."

—Robert Collier

CHAPTER 9

Your 7-Day CPAP Success Program

• • •

*"Progress comes slowly but steadily if you are
patient and prepare diligently."*

—JOHN WOODEN, LEGENDARY UCLA BASKETBALL COACH

BY NOW, YOU'RE PROBABLY FEELING overwhelmed with all of this information about CPAP and obstructive sleep apnea. You're pretty well versed in all the basic information, and eager to start making the necessary changes. You already have a CPAP machine, or you're waiting for it to be delivered. However, rather than becoming more hopeful about the prospect of getting a better night's sleep, you're more inclined to focus on the negatives. Now that you see this machine in front of you, you lose sight of your goal and instead ask yourself, "How am I ever going to get used to using this 'thing' every night for the rest of my life?" Just as any new health regimen seems daunting at the beginning, you may be asking yourself, "Where do I even start?"

This is the reaction that 99% of first-time CPAP users have at the beginning. Your emotions may override your logic and that 'resistance' may be starting to kick in. However, before you let your emotions get the better of you, there are some simple steps that will significantly increase your chances of success with CPAP.

I've broken down the steps into seven sections. You can plan on setting aside one day per step, just to make it more easily digestible. If you are progressing well, it's okay to combine some steps and finish in less than seven days, but it's important not to skip any of the steps.

I also recommend that you keep a sleep journal. Jot down things that you need to do, how well you slept during the night, how long you slept total and with the mask, how you feel in the morning after waking up, or any other CPAP issues you may have experienced. You can also jot down your basic CPAP adherence numbers from the machine, or any other information relevant to your care, such as discussions you had with your physician or DME company.

These seven steps also apply to those of you who are struggling with CPAP. Assuming you've addressed all the troubleshooting steps outlined in the previous chapters, you're ready to try once again.

There's an old adage that says, "What you don't measure, you can't manage." This applies whether your goal is to lose weight, make more money, or even improve your golf game. The same holds true for your CPAP success. The hardest part will be getting started.

Day 1: Education & Goal Setting

The more you understand what's really at stake here, the more reasons you'll have to keep going when the going gets tough. Get a clear picture in your mind as to what you'll miss out on if you were to let your sleep apnea go untreated. Perhaps it's the thought of not seeing your grandchildren grow up, or not being able to take time to travel around the world with your wife. Or, like one patient, seeing his friend who was THE model of success lose everything in an instant after suffering a stroke, then watching him being fed and changed like a helpless baby, and seeing him

98

confined to a wheelchair for the rest of his life. The clearer you get about why you need to address this potentially life-threatening condition, the more likely you are to succeed when you follow the steps outlined in this chapter. Write everything down on paper (or on your computer).

Day 2: Practice, Practice, Practice

Learning to live with CPAP is a temporarily challenging process that takes time for you to adapt and become acclimated. That being said, it doesn't have to disrupt your lifestyle. It's not like swallowing a pill, where you take one simple action and expect the pill to start working. In cases where patients are given CPAP with minimal counseling, education, and support, the chances of long-term success are relatively small.

Your first experience using CPAP may have been in the sleep lab. In this situation, you began using CPAP within one to two hours of being first introduced. The technician may have found the right CPAP pressure, but only had one night to make sure that you had the right mask that could be used over weeks, months and years. Ideally, you should be given your mask along with the necessary headgear, so you can practice wearing it long before you even receive your CPAP machine. If this is not an option, don't start using your machine right away. Spend the necessary time learning from your DME provider, whether in your home or in the sleep lab/DME facility, and ask any questions that you may have.

The first day or night, place the mask on your face as instructed and wear it for a few hours after dinner. Don't hook up the hose or connect it to the machine. Wear only the mask. Watch TV, work on the computer or read a book. Play Darth Vader with your kids. Leave it on until you go to bed. The purpose of this exercise is for you to get used to having something on your face, and still be able to focus on other activities without being distracted by the mask. If you have time to do this for short periods during the day, even better. Once you're comfortable with the mask, try sleeping with it, but don't connect it to the hose.

Day 3: Apply Pressure

On this evening, it's time to connect to your CPAP machine. After dinner, connect your mask to the machine and turn it on. Leave it on for 15 to 30 minutes and try to breathe naturally with the machine. If the ramp setting is on, turn it off or wait longer than the time it takes to increase the pressure to the prescribed levels. While it's on, watch TV, browse the Internet or read a book. I don't recommend that you eat while using CPAP. Try to do this again just before you go to sleep. You want to get to the point where you can lose yourself in your normal activities without being distracted by having a mask blowing air into your nose.

Trying to blow out against a constant pressure can feel strange. Some people think that it feels claustrophobic or that it creates feelings of anxiety. This is why it's important to begin this process slowly, in short intervals. Just like any new experience, with constant usage, most people do adapt and adjust.

This is also a good opportunity to experience what a leak feels like. With the machine running, open your mouth to see what it feels like to have a mouth leak. Move your mask around to create a leak. Play with the straps to feel what it's like to have them too loose or too tight. If you're up to it, take a short nap with the mask on.

Some people will need to do this for a few more days to reach the point of being comfortable and acclimated. You'll know when you're ready to move forward with this step. If you can't get past this step, it's time to call for professional help. It's also important to get the support of family and loved ones during this transition and trial period.

Day 4: Sleeping with CPAP

Continue the activities for Day 3. Put on your mask and turn on the machine for about 30 minutes before going to sleep, but this time, leave your machine on when you turn the lights out. If the mask comes off or if you wake up for any reason, readjust the mask and go back to sleep. If you have to go to the bathroom at night, disconnect your mask from the hose, but leave your mask on while you go to the bathroom. Remember that if you leave the machine running, it may record a large leak and also affect your adherence and therapy numbers. Some models can tell if you're not using the machine, even if you leave it on. If you use the ramp function, waking up to go to the bathroom can also affect your adherence data, and it will take time for you to reach your optimal pressure. Most experienced CPAP users will forego using the ramp function.

When you wake up the next morning, take note of how you slept. How often did you wake up? Was your mouth dry? Is the skin on your face or nose irritated? Was your sleep quality worse, the same or better than your usual night's sleep? If you slept well and had no problems whatsoever, keep doing what you're doing. If you had any problems during the night, take note of it and you can troubleshoot yourself, or call your DME or sleep physician to promptly address your concerns. Most machines will also have adherence data available, which you can use to troubleshoot.

Day 5: Troubleshooting

Most people will have one or more issues during their first few nights of sleep using CPAP. Go through the list of common problems in this book and follow the recommendations. Communicate with your DME or sleep physician ASAP. Most problems can be solved the next night by trying something different, but sometimes you may need to change the settings or order a part, so it may take a few extra days to resolve your problem.

Day 6: Modify and Try Again

I mentioned Einstein's quote earlier, which states that insanity is doing something over and over again but expecting different results. Trying CPAP again and again without making a change in what you're doing doesn't make sense. Based on what your problem is, read through the troubleshooting chapter again or call your DME company or sleep physician.

One simple option is to consider changing to a different mask. For example, if your nose is stuffy, then consider switching to a full-face mask that covers your nose and mouth.

If you're still at wits' end, your sleep laboratory may be able to offer you a formal CPAP desensitization program, with or without a PAP-NAP, which is a daytime CPAP titration nap study.

Day 7: CPAP Success

With persistence and some troubleshooting, most of you should be able to get measurably better sleep within the first week. For some of you, it may take a few more weeks or even months, but eventually, you can find solutions that work to improve your sleep. Then again, you may be one of the very few out there who will continue to struggle, no matter how many steps are taken.

If you're successful, don't think that it's going to continue forever. Guaranteed, sooner or later, you'll encounter problems with your CPAP machine or your sleep won't be as good as it used to be. There are a number of variables affecting the machine and you that are constantly changing, so it's important to have a routine maintenance schedule that you follow. I discussed CPAP cleaning routines in an earlier chapter. Just like your car, if you don't maintain your CPAP machine, it will not work properly.

At any point in this seven-day process, if you're not able to move on, go back a step or two or talk with your DME provider or sleep physician.

A good DME company should follow up with you frequently, especially in the first month, when getting you to use your machine and getting better sleep are so critical to long-term success. However, don't rely solely on your DME vendor. Assemble your 'dream team' and do it early on. Find a handful of providers who are easily accessible and will take the time to answer your questions. Most importantly, find a support group, whether with in-person AWAKE meetings (American Sleep Apnea Association) or online CPAP forums. Of course, you can do all this on your own – many of my patients have done so – but many more have told me that they would have quit their CPAP many times over if it hadn't been for the online support and camaraderie from those who were going through the same challenges as they were. I'll cover how to make these online connections in more detail in Chapter 10.

Every three to six months, you should also re-evaluate your sleep quality. With so many other stressors in life that can affect your sleep quality (new job, new children, weight gain, etc.), you may not immediately notice that your CPAP is not working as well as it did in the past. This is why it's important to write down how well you're sleeping in a sleep journal. For example, every six months, you can compare how you're feeling now to what you wrote six months ago. Are you more drowsy or tired in later afternoon meetings? Are you unable to stay focused while working? Are you snapping more often at your children or spouse?

Besides all the factors involved with CPAP, your general sleep hygiene and sleep habits will also contribute to your overall quality of sleep and how well rested you feel. To listen to an interview that I did with Dr. Shelby Harris on how to improve your sleep habits and hygiene, please visit doctorstevenpark.com/harris.

CHAPTER 10

Final Words

• • •

"Be not afraid of growing slowly, be afraid only of standing still."

—CHINESE PROVERB

CONGRATULATIONS ON READING THIS FAR. This means that you take your health seriously and are willing do whatever it takes to sleep better. Whenever I read a book, if I can take away one important point or concept that I can apply in my life with positive results, then it was worth reading. I hope that this book helped you as well. Hopefully, you got much more than one important point—perhaps even a revelation.

WHEN SHOULD YOU GIVE UP ON CPAP?

Bill is a middle-aged, slightly overweight lawyer who came to see me for surgical options. He tried three different types of CPAP machines (CPAP, bi-level PAP and APAP) with no significant improvement in his sleep. He also went through five different masks before finding that a full-face mask was comfortable enough to use. His sleep doctor had told him that his "numbers looked perfect" from his machine, with no more apneas (breathing pauses) and he was using 100% of the time without fail. However, despite meeting these objective criteria for CPAP success,

Bill subjectively felt that his sleep is much worse with his machine than without it.

For some of you, nothing works, no matter how much you try. You may have tried every suggestion in this book, including seven different masks, and three different PAP machines. You're even breathing better after nasal surgery, but still can't keep your CPAP mask on for more than one or two hours. Or, perhaps you are able to keep the mask on all night, with perfect compliance numbers and minimal AHI levels, but you still don't feel any better after six months.

Sleep physicians often talk about sleep debt. If you've had obstructive sleep apnea for years or decades, you won't feel better the first night or even within the first few weeks. Sometimes, it can take months to rebalance your 'sleep account' (assuming you're using CPAP). However, if you've gone through all the troubleshooting steps and you're not any better after many months, or if you're feeling worse, then it's time to have a discussion with your sleep physician about other options. Make sure that you don't have expiratory palatal obstruction or epiglottis collapse, which can prevent CPAP use (see sidebar, Chapter 6). Treating either of these two conditions surgically will not cure your sleep apnea completely, but may help you to tolerate CPAP or dental appliances more effectively.

When should you give up on CPAP? This is a difficult question to answer, since there are many different reasons why this happens, and everyone is different. However, after a certain point you have to say enough is enough. If good quality sleep is important to you, then you have to bite the bullet and move on to other options. The question is...which one?

OTHER OSA OPTIONS TO CONSIDER

The two other major options besides CPAP are dental appliances and surgery. Both of these options have plenty of good evidence-based research behind them, but only if applied properly. Dental options are numerous, and surgery has even more options, for different situations. A full discussion of both options are beyond the scope of this book. For more information about mandibular advancement devices, please listen to an interview with Dr. David Lawler at doctorstevenpark.com/lawler.

I also list a number of other resources from my website and outside sources of information in the resources chapter. The same goes for surgery alternatives, including a podcast titled "7 Good Reasons to Consider Surgery for Sleep Apnea," which you can find on doctorstevenpark.com. The most important question to ask before considering either of these options is—are you a good candidate? There are good published guidelines by various specialty societies that are great rules to follow, but an in-person evaluation by a qualified sleep surgeon is always best. You can find recommendations regarding mandibular advancement devices[1] and surgery[2] published by the American Academy of Sleep Medicine in the reference section at the end of this book.

I also extensively list alternative and complementary options in the resources section. This includes my take on tongue exercises, acupuncture, Provent®, and the didgeridoo (an Australian Aborigine musical instrument).

Bill ultimately decided to undergo nasal surgery to improve his nasal congestion. During the procedure, an examination of his airways during deep sleep revealed that his soft palate was backing up into his nose, causing sudden blockages in breathing during mid-nasal exhalation. This was addressed in a separate procedure with a conservative palate operation, which allowed him to use CPAP much more effectively. Although he's not sleeping like he did in his 20s, his sleep quality is now improved enough for him to function much better at work and enjoy life again.

In my experience, most people find significant relief after undergoing one round of targeted surgery, whereas others will need additional surgery.

Some people end up effectively using CPAP with a dental appliance after nasal surgery. One is not ever better than another. You need to choose an option that makes sense to you (as long as it's medically appropriate), and try your best to make it work. However, don't get stuck on just one form of therapy or its variations.

Also, consider trying mandibular advancement devices or even targeted surgery to augment the other options. For example, Bill's nasal and palate procedures not only allowed him to breathe better through his nose, but also allowed his CPAP pressure to decrease significantly, which made it much more comfortable for him, with a lower likelihood of mask leaks.

> **Will A Mandibular Advancement Device Work For Me?**
>
> Only a certified sleep dentist can tell you whether you're a good candidate, but one thing that I strongly recommend to check for before getting fitted for a dental appliance is to undergo a quick office endoscopy by an otolaryngologist (ENT surgeon). It's important to make sure that your tongue and soft palate open up significantly as you thrust your lower jaw forward. This should be done while lying flat on your back with your head in a neutral position (not too tilted forward or cocked back). For see a video of this procedure, please see the resources section (Nasal endoscopy video example).

The Importance of an Online Community

As much as I emphasize the basic fundamentals when using CPAP, I can't emphasize enough how important it is to search for and rely on your online support community. These valuable resources can be found on a number of sites, including CPAPtalk.com and Hope2SleepGuide. As I stated in the beginning of this book, interacting with and learning from thousands of people on these support sites formed the basic foundations of my own knowledge base. Please see the resources chapter for a more complete list. Not only can you find people who want to help, but many of these people have also gone through precisely what you're experiencing. You may also find a connection with one or two trustworthy individuals with whom you can communicate offline.

One word of caution, however. As with any online source of information, including comments or reviews, you have to take everything with a grain of salt. These people are not dispensing medical advice. You'll also have occasional naysayers, discouraging you from trying something different based on their own negative experiences, even though research papers and other experts hold a different opinion. Others will tell you to keep trying, despite the fact that you've tried to the best of your ability for years. What the online community can give you is emotional and community support, which medical professionals are usually not able to provide.

Follow Your Own CPAP Data

Once you start using CPAP, there's a lot of paperwork happening behind the scenes to make sure that you're using your PAP machine appropriately. For certain insurance companies that require this, you'll have to show the DME that you're compliant (see the CPAP Stickiness chapter). In most situations, your adherence data is stored on a small SD card in the back of the machine. This data is downloaded by your DME periodically during the first three months. This can happen manually during a face-to-face visit, or during a visit with your sleep lab or physician. Another option is to use Wi-Fi to send data automatically to your CPAP-ordering physician. With this feature, the physician can remotely change your pressure or settings based on the data that's visible securely online. Either way, it can be an arduous process, with lots of faxes, correspondences, and phone calls.

In order to be proactive and track your own data, download and install a program called SleepyHead to look at your own data. You'll need a computer that can read SD cards. This software can read most modern PAP machines, and it prints the data out in a much more reader-friendly format than the conventional software that manufacturers provide to DMEs and sleep labs. If you're not computer savvy, then a family member or friend can help you with the initial set-up process. It's a way of preemptively troubleshooting any potential problems and giving immediate feedback to your sleep physician, who can then make the necessary adjustments. Nowadays, many CPAP manufacturers also have online programs that serve similar functions.

There are a number of different variables that are reported, but the three main numbers to look at are average AHI, average leak rates, and total hours used every night. You want your AHI to be very low (much less than five) every night, with very low leak rates, and you want to be using CPAP for at least four hours every night. Based on these numbers and how well you sleep at night, you can troubleshoot any other problems that may arise.

For example, if you were sleeping very well for months, but very poorly for the last three nights, you may find that you're having some large leaks and your AHI is higher than normal, but the total hours of use have not changed. You realize that you caught a cold three days ago and your nose has been stuffy. It's likely that you opened your mouth to breathe at night, which caused a mouth leak. To solve this problem, you can simply give it a few more days for the cold to go away, or you can decongest your nose with nasal saline. A more aggressive option is to use an over-the-counter 12-hour decongestant spray (oxymetazoline, or Afrin®), along with nasal dilator strips. Again, if you do use Afrin®, it's important not to use it for more than three days in a row, since you can easily become addicted to it.

If the mouth leak is a chronic problem and you're breathing well through your nose, two other options are to add a chin strap (to help keep your mouth closed) or to switch from your nasal mask to a full-face mask. It's also likely that you'll feel the leaks when they occur, since it causes the CPAP pressure to go down and your apneas to increase, leading to obstruction and arousal.

As mentioned before, the most pro-active and resourceful patients are those that see the best results with CPAP.

KEEP COPIES OF YOUR SLEEP STUDIES WITH YOU

If you've ever looked at a sleep study report, it can be a 10-page maze of numbers and squiggly lines. There's usually a summary page in the front or near the end, but even that can be confusing and packed with technical terminology. When ordering CPAP, the DMEs usually look for the original diagnostic AHI and the date of the study. For a CPAP titration, they need the CPAP pressure and the date. Oftentimes, patients never see the full report, since they are simply told what the results are.

However, it's a good idea to get copies of the full report for your records. If you change sleep doctors, or need to see a dentist or a surgeon for consultation, then you'll need the latest copies. Sometimes, your DME closes down, your insurance changes or your doctor retires. In all these situations, you may need quick access to your latest sleep study results.

BREATHE BETTER, SLEEP BETTER, LIVE BETTER

My initial goal in writing this book was to provide you with THE most comprehensive resource on CPAP. This would have ended up being over 300 pages – not something I'd inflict on my medical residents, let alone those of you who are most likely sleep deprived! Instead, I decided to give you a practical, easy-to-read book that can give you quick results. As I've mentioned before, this book is not meant to be a substitute for a face-to-face interaction with your sleep physician or DME provider. However, I hope that what you learned from reading this book will form the basic knowledge base that you'll need to have efficient and meaningful discussions with your healthcare providers.

More importantly, I hope that you'll be able to take the initiative to take action and keep making forward progress. Remember, your resourcefulness can be just as important, if not more important, than your available resources. All of the people mentioned in this book (Jason, Suzy, Louise, Jonathan, Peter and Bill) had the right resources, but relied on their resourcefulness to keep asking questions and never giving up until their CPAP problems were solved.

By taking charge of your own healthcare decisions and knowing who or what to ask for, you'll be much more likely to see improvements in how well you sleep using CPAP.

Lastly, having the right resources and resourcefulness will not make any difference if you do not have the right mindset from the very beginning. Why do you need to get optimal sleep? For your family, your children, for school or for your career? Do you have any of the objections outlined in Chapter 4? Are you willing to deal with these self-limiting beliefs?

Hopefully, you found this book to be helpful for your journey to better sleep and a better life. Armed with the right mindset, along with the resources provided in this book, you'll have the resourcefulness to finally restore your sleep and reclaim your life.

A Favor to Ask of You

If you found the information in this book helpful, I would truly appreciate any feedback from you. If you have any comments or suggestions, or if you disagree with me about anything, please feel free contact me directly at doctorpark@doctorstevenpark.com.

Also, if you enjoyed the book, or found it helpful, I would also appreciate a positive review on this book's Amazon page, so that others like you can benefit from this book. Last but not least, if you have other topics you'd like for me to cover in more detail, please let me know. Lastly, browse through the resources chapter as well as my website doctorstevenpark.com for more information.

• • •

Also online at totallycpap.com/resources

ONLINE RESOURCES

Doctorstevenpark.com. My blog with a wealth of information on obstructive sleep apnea, upper airway resistance syndrome, and various treatment options. Listen to my podcast here, or on iTunes (Breathe Better, Sleep Better, Live Better Podcast).

Sleepeducation.org. A sleep health information resource by the American Academy of Sleep Medicine

Entnet.org. American Academy of Otolaryngology – Head & Neck Surgery's patient health page listing various ENT health conditions

CPAPTalk.com. A vibrant online CPAP community

Sleeptember.org. American Sleep Apnea Association's site with lots of great resources

Hope2sleepguide.com. Helpful online sleep apnea-oriented forum

CPAP Resources

Freecpapadvice.com. A helpful site with lots of videos made by a registered polysomnographic sleep technician (RPST).

Hope2sleep.co.uk. A UK based charity with a wealth of information about OSA.

Padacheek.com. A variety of CPAP mask accessories, and strap pads and hose liners that make using CPAP more pleasant.

CPAP hose holders. Bruce Stein's book, *Sleep Apnea & CPAP: A User's Manual By A User*, describes an inexpensive way of suspending your hose. More convenient options can be purchased online.

Mandibular Advancement Devices. Find a certified dentist from the American Academy of Dental Sleep Medicine (aadsm.org).

Alternative Nonsurgical Options with Published Data

Myofunctional Therapy (tongue exercises). This study found a 50% drop in average AHI levels. It can be helpful in many patients. Find a certified myofunctional therapist. (https://tonguethrust.com/wp-content/uploads/2016/10/2015-Meta-Analysis-OSA-Myo-Rx..pdf)

Acupuncture. This study found about a 50% drop in average AHI scores with significant subjective improvement. If you're interested, take a copy of the paper's protocol with you to your local acupuncturist. (http://www.hsp.epm.br/dfisio/fisioneuro/afreire_sleepmedice2007.pdf)

Didgeridoo. A study found about a 50% drop in AHI levels with significant subjective improvement. (http://www.bmj.com/content/332/7536/266)

Provent. Novel disposable adhesive covers for your nostrils that provide mild resistance during nasal exhalation. (proventtherapy.com)

Other Options

Sleep Positioners. There are a number of different ways to keep you off your back. The simplest is to sew a tennis ball inside a sock to the back of your pajamas, but this is often too small to keep you off your back. Better options include devices by Rematee, ZZoma, and Slumberbump.

Wedges and other devices to elevate the top of your head can also help with obstructive sleep apnea and acid reflux. Reflux Guard is one such example.

There are countless other options that tout success in treating obstructive sleep apnea. I have no doubt that these options may work to varying degrees, but I have limited describing only options that have proven research data, or those that I found helpful for my patients.

Videos

Expiratory palatal obstruction (EPO). An example video of the soft palate flopping back into the nose during mid-nasal exhalation. This can prevent CPAP or dental appliance use. It can also present as central apneas since there's no airflow through the nose and mouth, and no movement of the abdomen and chest. (http://doctorstevenpark.com/epo)

Epiglottis collapse. An example of the epiglottis flopping back during inhalation. This can also prevent CPAP or dental appliance use. It's important to note that both EPO and epiglottis collapse can occur without any significant apneas seen in a sleep study. (http://doctorstevenpark.com/epiglottis)

Nasal endoscopy video example. This is a short video of an endoscopic exam performed in the office. Initially, it's with the patient sitting up after topical nasal decongestion and anesthesia. You can see the right and left nasal anatomy, and the Mueller's maneuver in the middle of the video. Near the end, the patient is lying flat on her back, and you can see that the space behind the tongue base and epiglottis is much more narrow. At the very end, I have the patient thrust her lower jaw forward, which pulls the tongue base forward significantly, allowing you to see the voice box more clearly. This is one maneuver I do to determine if a patient is potentially a good candidate for a mandibular advancement device. (http://doctorstevenpark.com/nasalendoscopy)

Surgery for Obstructive Sleep Apnea

The Truth About Obstructive Sleep Apnea Surgery. Free e-book at doctorstevenpark.com/osasurgery).

REFERENCES

• • •

Chapter 1: Mastering the Fundamentals of CPAP

1. Nilius, G, et al. Pressure-relief continuous positive airway pressure vs. constant continuous positive airway pressure: a comparison of efficacy and compliance. *CHEST Journal* 130.4 (2006): 1018-1024.

Chapter 5: CPAP Stickiness

1. Weaver TE, Maislin G, Dinges DF, et al. Relationship Between Hours of CPAP Use and Achieving Normal Levels of Sleepiness and Daily Functioning. *Sleep.* 2007;30(6):711.

2. Weaver TE, Grunstein RR. Adherence to Continuous Positive Airway Pressure Therapy: The Challenge to Effective Treatment. *Proceedings of the American Thoracic Society.* 2008;5(2):173–178.

3. Engleman HM, Wild MR. Improving CPAP use by patients with the sleep apnoea/hypopnoea syndrome (SAHS). *Sleep Med Rev.* 2003;7(1):81–99.

4. Budhiraja R, Parthasarathy S, Drake CL, et al. Early CPAP use identifies subsequent adherence to CPAP therapy. *Sleep.* 2007;30(3):320–324.

5. Sin DD, Mayers I, Man GC, & Pawluk L. (2002). Long-term compliance rates to continuous positive airway pressure in obstructive sleep apnea: a population-based study. *CHEST Journal, 121*(2), 430-435.

6. Krieger J, Kurtz, D, Petiau C, Sforza E, & Trautmann D. (1996). Long-term compliance with CPAP therapy in obstructive sleep apnea patients and in snorers. *Sleep, 19*(9 Suppl), S136-43.

7. Campos-Rodríguez F, Martínez-García MA, Reyes-Núñez N, Almeida-González CV, Catalán-Serra P, & Montserrat J. M. (2012). Long-term CPAP compliance in women with obstructive sleep apnoea. *European Respiratory Journal, 40*(Suppl 56), P434.

8. Stepnowsky CJ, & Dimsdale JE. (2002). Dose–response relationship between CPAP compliance and measures of sleep apnea severity. *Sleep medicine, 3*(4), 329-334.

9. McArdle N, Devereux G, Heidarnejad H, Engleman HM, Mackay TW, & Douglas NJ. (1999). Long-term use of CPAP therapy for sleep apnea/hypopnea syndrome. *American Journal of Respiratory and Critical Care Medicine, 159*(4), 1108-1114.

10. Poirier J, George C, Rotenberg B. The effect of nasal surgery on nasal continuous positive airway pressure compliance. *Laryngoscope.* 2014;124(1):317–319.

Chapter 6: Your Top 15 CPAP Problems, Solved

1 The use of bisphenol A in manufacture of ResMed CPAP Devices. www.resmed.com/cn/assets/documents/service_support/faq/20110505105800276.pdf.

2. Watson NF, Sue KM. Aerophagia and gastroesophageal reflux disease in patients using continuous positive airway pressure: a preliminary observation. JCSM 2008;4(5):434.

3. Simmons JH. Treating aerophagia-induced gastric distress (AIGD) associated with CPAP therapy to improve CPAP outcome: Understanding the relationship behind oral pressure leakage and AIGD development is key to treatment success. Sleep 2014 Abstract Supplement. Vol. 37:A108.

4. Quan, SF, Budhiraja R, Clarke DP, Goodwin JL, Gottlieb, DJ, Nichols DA, & Kushida CA. (2013). Impact of treatment with continuous positive airway pressure (CPAP) on weight in obstructive sleep apnea. *Journal of clinical sleep medicine: JCSM: official publication of the American Academy of Sleep Medicine*, *9*(10), 989.

CHAPTER 7: MORE HELPFUL CPAP TIPS

1. Passengers with CPAPs, BiPaps, and APAPs. https://www.tsa.gov/contact/customer-service.

CHAPTER 10: FINAL WORDS

1. http://www.aasmnet.org/Resources/clinicalguidelines/Oral_appliance-OSA.pdf

2. http://www.aasmnet.org/Resources/PracticeParameters/PP_SurgicalModificationsOSA.pdf

ACKNOWLEDGEMENTS

• • •

ALTHOUGH A SMALLER PROJECT THAN my prior book, *Sleep, Interrupted*, this book required the same amount of effort and involvement by countless people. An enormous amount of gratitude goes to all my patients and those with whom I interacted on my website and various online communities.

In particular, I wish to thank the initial reviewers who gave me the valuable perspectives and important suggestions that made this an infinitely better book: David Levine, Claire Powers, Claudia Storonskij, and Chip Smith from Restoration Medical Supply.

Also, a big note of thanks to my editors Dianne Purdie and Happy Marli. Thank you for your patience and constructive comments and suggestions, which made the manuscript so much more readable.

Most of all, I want to thank my publisher Jodev Press for putting up with my endless delays and revisions.

ABOUT THE AUTHOR

• • •

DR. STEVEN Y. PARK IS an author, blogger, speaker and surgeon with a passion for educating the lay public about the importance of good breathing while sleeping for optimal health. He is the author of the Amazon bestseller, *Sleep Interrupted: A physician reveals the #1 reason why so many of us are sick and tired*, which was endorsed by numerous New York Times best-selling authors, including Dr. Christiane Northrup, Dr. Mark Liponis, Dr. Dean Ornish and Ms. Mary Shomon.

His blog has been rated one of the "Best Sleep Disorder Blogs of 2016" by Healthline.com, Best of Doctor Websites 2106 by Pacific Medical Training, and a "Top 10 online influencer of sleep discussion" by Sharecare.com.

Dr. Park has been quoted in the New York Times, Forbes, Scientific American, Parade Magazine, Woman's World, WebMD, Glamour, Huffington Post, US News, and MSN Health, among others.

He is board-certified in both otolaryngology and sleep medicine, and is also an Assistant Professor of Otorhinolaryngology at the Albert Einstein College of Medicine.

For more information about Dr. Park, please visit www.doctorstevenpark.com.